Contemporar

Ballet

AUDREY
WILLIAMSON

Contemporary
Ballet

DA CAPO PRESS · NEW YORK · 1980

Library of Congress Cataloging in Publication Data

Williamson, Audrey, 1913-
    Contemporary ballet.

    (Da Capo series in dance)
    Reprint of the 1946 ed. published by Rockliff,
London.
    1. Ballet. 2. Modern dance. I. Title.
GV1787.W55 1980   792.8   80-16224
ISBN 0-306-76041-X

This Da Capo Press edition of
Contemporary Ballet is an unabridged
republication of the first edition
published in London in 1946
by Rockliff Publishing Company.

Published by Da Capo Press, Inc.
A Subsidiary of Plenum Publishing Corporation
227 West 17th Street, New York, N.Y. 10011

CONTEMPORARY BALLET

FOR

ROBERT HELPMANN

IN APPRECIATION OF HIS INVALUABLE
WORK FOR SADLER'S WELLS AS DANCER
AND MIME, AND THE COURAGE AND
IMAGINATION WITH WHICH, AS A
CHOREOGRAPHER, HE HAS GIVEN A NEW
DIRECTION TO CONTEMPORARY BALLET

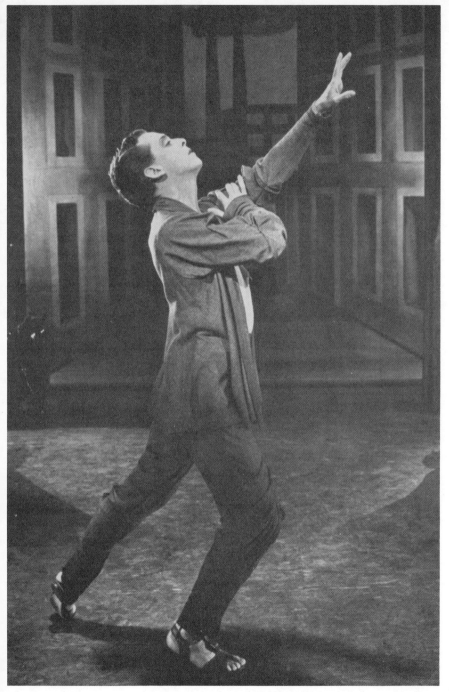

Photo   Edward Mandinian

"Line" in Modern Ballet
Robert Helpmann in *Miracle in the Gorbals*

Plate I

AUDREY

WILLIAMSON

Contemporary

Ballet

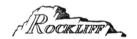

SALISBURY SQUARE · LONDON

1946

PRINTED BY
WATMOUGHS LIMITED, IDLE, BRADFORD;
AND LONDON

CONTENTS

LIST OF PLATES

LIST OF PLATES

LIST OF PLATES

INTRODUCTION

THIS book makes no attempt to be a ballet history or to give a detailed analysis of the Russian ballets which were seen in England during the period before the war. The scene has been fully covered by critics who wrote while the ballets and performances were fresh in their minds; the companies as they were then composed are no longer in existence, and of the development of the Russian dancers during the past six years it is impossible for the English critic to write with authority. The main emphasis of this book, therefore, is inevitably on the work of the companies performing within this country during and immediately after the war period, but I have at the same time tried to give a comprehensive study of more general aspects of ballet as an art and in this the important achievements of Russian Ballet, modern and classical, fall into their proper place.

I wish particularly to thank Mr. P. J. S. Richardson and Miss Frances Stephens, editors of *The Dancing Times* and *Theatre World*, for permission to use material from articles and reviews which appeared originally in their magazines, Miss Joan Lawson for her help in several ways, and Mme Vera Volkova for her kindness in allowing me to attend her private classes. I am also grateful to Mr. George Bernard Shaw for permission to print an extract from his book, *Music in London*, 1890–1894 (Constable), and to Mr. Cyril Beaumont for similar permission to quote from his admirable translations of Noverre's *Lettres sur la Danse et les Ballets* and of Gautier's writings in his publication, *The Romantic Ballet as seen by Théophile Gautier*. I should also like to thank Mme Nadine Nicolaeva-Legat for allowing me to use extracts from her late husband's book, *Ballets Russes* (Methuen), and to visit her school and classes; also my good friend Mr. G. B. L. Wilson for his kindness in compiling the Index.

Finally, to all the photographers who have collaborated to produce such a fine pictorial record of ballet I wish to extend my most grateful acknowledgment, particularly in the case of Mr. Gordon Anthony, who found negatives for me while on leave from the R.A.F., and Mr. G. B. L. Wilson, Miss Peggy Delius and Mr. Roger Wood, whose action photographs are interesting examples of a branch of photography requiring exceptional skill and patience.

AUDREY WILLIAMSON.

London. May 1946.

GENERAL ASPECTS

CHAPTER I

HISTORY AND DEVELOPMENT

THE history of ballet as an art is a history of its struggle for dramatic expression as apart from mere display and technical virtuosity. It is imperative that this is realised if ballet is to maintain any intellectual hold on the imagination and the high rank as an art of the theatre which many educated people, unaware of its dramatic and poetic range of expression, still deny to it.

Ballet as a professional art of the theatre dates from 1661, when Louis XIV founded the Académie Royale de Danse, an institution which still exists and flourishes in Paris. Prior to this it had been primarily a Court spectacle, introduced into France from Italy by Catherine de Medici, performed by amateurs of the aristocracy (Louis XIV himself was an enthusiastic dancer who for many years executed the leading rôles in all important Court ballets), and acting either as the equivalent of a firework display at Court fêtes or as a spectacular diversion, normally including singing and poetry, at banquet celebrations. Obviously at such functions the principal objects would be entertainment and pageantry, making as few mental demands as possible on the noble but possibly already soporific guests, and there is a modern parallel in our night club "dinner and cabaret"; although the entertainments of the French Court at the height of the glory of the "Sun King" must far have exceeded their degenerate modern counterpart in lavishness and artistic taste.

The founding of an Academy of the Dance, however, set ballet free to develop along more serious lines in the theatre instead of the Court, made possible the development of dance technique through systematically trained professional dancers, and finally gave to the art a freedom of movement, brilliance and aerial quality which had never been possible in the old Court ballets, composed purely in terms of geometrical pattern and chained to the ground by the amateur status of the dancer and the long skirts and heavy inadaptability of contemporary costume. Yet in this very enrichment of the technical

3

vocabulary of the dance, and concentration on the virtuosity of individual dancers, lay a danger for the future; and costume reform, although given its first stimulus by Camargo's shortening of the skirt by six inches in about 1730, and Sallé's courageous attempt in the same decade to introduce a costume appropriate in period to her Greek part of Galatea, was still far from complete. If it was King Louis's Academy which first made ballet possible as an artistic entity, working on a professional basis within the theatre, it was the publication in 1760, almost exactly a century later, of Noverre's *Lettres sur la Danse et les Ballets* which first made ballet articulate, and set forth the ideal of ballet as a dramatic and expressive art in a book which remains to this day the most valuable and clear-sighted exposition of ballet as an art and the dancer as an artist. Noverre in his book also, though with less success, vigorously attacked the conventional masks, pannier skirts, elaborate wigs and dress ornamentation that restricted expression and movement in the ballets of his time, much as his great successor Fokine, a hundred and fifty years later, revolted against the period inaccuracies of costume in the Russian Imperial Ballet.

Jean George Noverre was the most distinguished composer of ballets (or in our modern term choreographer) of his time, a dancer (as all choreographers have been) and famous as a creator of the *ballet d'action*, the form of ballet in which the dancing is used not as an end in itself but to illustrate a dramatic story. The idea of drama expressed through dance was not a new one. A thread of plot narration, the story of Circe, was introduced into the celebrated *Ballet Comique de la Reine*, probably the first ballet as we understand the term, produced in 1581 by Catherine de Medici's valet, the violinist Beaujoyeux, to celebrate the betrothal of the Duc de Joyeuse and Marguerite de Lorraine; and dance as a form of dramatic expression dates back to the Roman mime plays and to the theatres of ancient Greece, where dance and mimed gesture were incorporated into the plays of Æschylus and Sophocles as a visual illustration of the poetry, and where the art was held in esteem as an essential part of Greek culture. Aristotle's definition of dancing as "the representation of actions, characters and passions by means of postures and rhythmic movements" is some indication of its expressive use at this time. But Noverre was the first to create ballet deliberately as a dramatic and artistic entity and to analyse its full potentialities in words. And his quality as artist and thinker may be gauged by the fact that Voltaire wrote in his praise and Garrick, whose naturalness and versatility as an actor Noverre set down in his book as the ideal for dancers to follow, named him "the Shakespeare of the Dance." He was the first great reformer of ballet and it is significant that ballet reform has always come from within, through the practical artists of the theatre and never through the writing or theorising of the *littérateur* and balletomane; though this has sometimes been of definite value for the propagation of new principles and movements already at work within the theatre, or forgotten from the past, and as a descriptive record of the dancers and ballets of a particular period. (Théophile Gautier, the French poet and critic of last century and librettist of the oldest ballet extant, the 100-year-old *Giselle*, comes into this last category as a vivid recorder of the Romantic period of ballet and a writer, like his prototype Lamb in the drama, of permanent literary value. Two ballet critics nearer our own time, the Russian Svetloff and French André Levinson, have also notably contributed to the art in this way.)

Carlo Blasis, the most erudite choreographer and dancer in ballet history and an early director of the Milan Academy of Dancing, founded in 1813 (the studies in which he excelled included music, drawing, painting, modelling, architecture, geometry, anatomy, literature and dancing, the knowledge of all of which he declared to be of assistance in the creation of ballet!), further emphasised Noverre's theories in his two most famous books, *Treatise on the Art of Dancing* and *The Code of Terpsichore*, but his special contribution to the dance was his exhaustive codifying of dance technique, which he enriched by the invention of at least one beautiful pose, the *attitude*, borrowed from Bologne's statue of Mercury. His system of dance training is still followed in Milan and has influenced ballet in every country, though it is now generally recognised that its exclusive use is unwise for the full artistic development of the dancer and it needs to be balanced by training in the softer and more extended Russian school. It is, however, the great choreographer of our own time, Fokine, who stands out in ballet history beside Noverre as a reformer of similar character who put his theories clearly and decisively into words; though it is of melancholy significance that like Noverre himself he had to leave his own country to carry out his principles to their full extent, an opportunity fortunately provided by his appointment as choreographer to the Russian Ballet company formed and brought to Europe by Diaghileff, with epoch-making results.

Noverre's *Letters on Dancing and Ballets* and Fokine's "five principles of ballet" laid down in a letter to *The Times* on 6th July 1914 are both an expression of revolt against the rigid tradition, mechanically applied and jealously fostered by balletomanes and critics, which had cramped the development of ballet in their time. In both cases the cry is the same, for the elimination of virtuosity for its own sake and the substitution of movement completely expressive of theme, character and story. Fokine, writing a century and a half after Noverre, echoes his predecessor not only in general ideas but also at moments in practically the same words. Most important of all, these are not mere theories, the abstract ideals of critics with no practical working knowledge of ballet; they are the self-explanation of the two greatest figures in the history of ballet, men who were already putting these ideas into practice and whose work has had a revolutionary influence on the whole trend of choreography.

The warning note here is obvious. The fact that Noverre's basic principles had to be reasserted little more than a century after his death emphasises the constant liability of ballet to degenerate as an art. This degeneracy invariably occurs under the same conditions, excessive concentration on the executant and the virtuosity of dance steps and arrangements, and its seed is inherent in the material of ballet itself. The appeal of ballet being primarily to the eye, there is a constant danger of the art degenerating into spectacle for its own sake, and of the audience contenting itself with looking and ceasing to think. "It is shameful," wrote Noverre, "that dancing should renounce the empire it might assert over the mind and only endeavour to please the sight." Fokine's "five principles" are the contemporary bulwark against this decadence, and their influence on ballet is still so extensive that they are worth summarising briefly even though they are now fairly generally known.

(1) The creation of dance styles appropriate to the subject of each ballet, and expressive of the period and nation represented.

(2) Dancing and mimetic gesture have no meaning in ballet unless they serve as an expression of its dramatic action, and they must not be used as a mere *divertissement* or entertainment, having no connection with the scheme of the whole ballet.

(3) The elimination of conventional gesture and sign language, except where required by the style of the ballet, and the replacing of gestures of the hands by mimetic of the whole body. "*Man can be and should be expressive from head to foot.*"

(4) Expressiveness in groups and ensemble dancing, so that the

dancers are not arranged in symmetrical groups purely for ornament, but to express whatever sentiment the action or theme requires.

(5) Complete equality between choreographer, designer and musician. Music and design not to be an "accompaniment" to the dance dictated by the choreographer, but an integral part of the whole ballet, artist and composer being given complete liberty in creation.

The result of Fokine's reforms was to set ballet free from the tyranny of hack "ballet" music, the ballerina's "tutu" skirt and pink satin slipper, the "dance *divertissement*" introduced for its own sake without any reference to the progression of the story, and all the other encumbrances which had become frozen, in nineteenth-century Russia, into a formula and brought ballet in England and the Continent, where there were no dance creators comparable to those in Russia, to a still lower level. It opened up to the choreographer a much wider range of subject matter and dance styles, and gave ballet an artistic integrity which placed it for the first time on a comparable level, as Noverre and Blasis had dreamed, with its sister arts of music, painting, literature and the drama. In the Diaghileff Ballet it produced a series of ballets of widely varying styles in which Fokine had as collaborators artists of the stature of Bakst, Benois and Roerich and, where existing music of high quality was not used, a young composer of the stature of Stravinsky. The ballets ranged from the romantic classical *Sylphides*, *Carnaval* and *Spectre de la Rose* to the exotic drama of *Scheherazade;* from the symbolic dance tragedy of a Russian puppet show, *Petrouchka*, to the virile and barbaric *Prince Igor*, which in its superb orchestration of male character dancing came as a revelation in Europe, where the male dancer had, at best, degenerated to a "ballerina's prop" and, at worst, been replaced by women *en travesti*. This was the peak period of Russian Ballet creation, and the pivot was Fokine with his conception of dance as a dramatic, musical and decorative whole.

How, in this light, do we stand to-day? Fokine is dead, and his greatest and most revolutionary work a quarter of a century old. Massine, under Diaghileff and later de Basil, has enriched the mechanism of the dance in a number of ballets that are complete works of art and some more, the symphonic ballets, that may remarkably influence technique but offer no line of development as artistic entities, since they add little or nothing to, and even in some cases (notably the

Beethoven) detract from, the music on which they are based. In England, Ninette de Valois has created at least one great work of dramatic and essentially English idiom, *The Rake's Progress*, and Frederick Ashton, more international in style, some beautiful and witty dance inventions culminating, early in the war, in two "abstract" ballets of outstanding technique, musicality and spiritual suggestion, *Dante Sonata* and *The Wanderer*. In America, more recently, a young English choreographer, Antony Tudor (working under conditions unaffected by the war), has produced a psychological dance drama, *Pillar of Fire*, which has been sensationally hailed as a masterpiece, not the least by some English critics who have not yet seen it; but the full originality and merit of this and other ballets produced in America since the war—by Tudor, the Russian Nijinska, Massine and Balanchine, and the American Agnes de Mille—as well as those by the choreographers of Soviet Russia, it is obviously not yet possible for us to gauge.

Of more immediate concern in England is the emergence of Robert Helpmann, a dancer-mime of considerable talent and experience, as a choreographer who in less than five years of ballet creation has produced three great works which continue the dramatic trend given to English ballet by Ninette de Valois, and suggest interesting new lines of development. *Hamlet*, produced in 1942 within six months of Helpmann's first ballet, *Comus*, is a work of driving imagination in which dance, mime, music and *décor*, as in Fokine's ideal, are superbly welded. Its originality lies in its free merging of dance with dramatic gesture and movement, and its use of ballet as a psychological illumination, through the fourth dimension of a dream, of a work of art in another medium. *Miracle in the Gorbals*, produced two years later, develops this individual and dramatic form of dance (neither ballet makes use of "pointwork" or conventional classic technique, though their emphasis on "line" has a classic foundation) and is a first attempt by ballet in this country to use a realistic modern scene and characters as a comment on slum conditions. With *Adam Zero*, Helpmann's instinct for the alliance of stage production and dance has reached a new and original phase of development. Combining an expressionistic theatre technique with a flexible and complex use of groups and dance forms, this ballet reveals the new possibilities open to the choreographer on the Covent Garden stage, and the moving power and beauty an allegory may attain through the ballet medium. It is an *Everyman* of our own time, as contemporary in spirit as *Miracle in the Gorbals* but more timeless and poetic in construction and implication.

All Helpmann's ballets are magnificent "theatre," a term which has been applied to *Hamlet* as a reproach. Such a view curiously ignores the fact that ballet is essentially and by tradition an art of the theatre, and the ballet which is good theatre is more likely to be a good ballet than the ballet which is not. Noverre, Viganò, Blasis and Fokine, the greatest creators of the past, all recognised this, and it is in English ballet to-day that their conception of ballet as an art with *meaning*, combining pantomime and dance to present characters, stories and (a later development) symbolic ideas, shows signs of being most productively developed. And just because the dramatic experiments of Helpmann and equally theatrical character ballets of Ninette de Valois are balanced by Ashton's expressive use of purer dance forms and the preservation in the same repertoire of the Russian classical ballets, natural evolution is unlikely to become twisted into a revolutionary blind alley. No one realised better than Fokine the necessity of building on the foundation of the past, with the result that Fokine's creations live to-day as the basis for further developments, while the purely individual and self-expressional dance of Isadora Duncan survives only as an influence on dance and not in any concrete form. Her most constructive influence has been on the classical ballet she derided, for Fokine in his youth saw her and was influenced by her theories on music and period "style," which he freely adapted into the larger framework of ballet.

Ballet throughout its history has shown this facility to select and absorb from every form of dance, and though every reformer has been bitterly opposed by the conservative (the outcry of some self-styled custodians of the dance at Helpmann's *Hamlet* was merely an echo across the years of that of Russian balletomanes at the production of Fokine's early ballet *Eunice*, created under the influence of Duncan's Grecian style of dance and costume), in the long run it is seen that these reforms, being conceived within ballet and not outside it, have their roots in solid ground, and so far from destroying ballet enrich and renew it for succeeding generations. Ballet is in danger not when it uses its dance for dramatic ends but when such ends are forgotten and dramatic expression opposed in the name of "dance for the sake of dance." This is the lesson that Noverre and Fokine have taught us, and that ballet, in England and elsewhere, must continue to follow if it is to have mind and passion as well as beauty.

CHAPTER II

THE ART OF CHOREOGRAPHY

THIS quality of mind, a recognised criterion of greatness in the writer, the artist and the composer, is an element in choreography to which a large proportion of balletgoers seem indifferent. Yet it is of prime importance in establishing true values as distinct from degrees of technical facility, and without it the artist will merely skim the surface of his medium and the texture of paint, words, dance or music lack the spiritual depth and richness of the true master.

It is a quality difficult to define, instinctive rather than consciously produced, and only in the writer and poet can it be recognised through the literal analysis of thought and idea. Imagination, originality, emotional and spiritual content, all these are a part of it, and it is obvious that in ballet, as in the novel and the play, the choice of subject will limit or release its expression. It is recognisable in Shakespeare through *Hamlet* and *King Lear* rather than *Much Ado About Nothing* and *Love's Labour's Lost*, in Fokine through *Petrouchka*, the symbolic tragedy of humanity, the puppet with a soul, groping towards love and self-expression, rather than the ballroom flirtations of *Carnaval* and the shallow prettiness of *Les Elfes*. It marks the great work, which is rare, from the charming or brilliant, in which ballet has been prolific. Very few choreographers possess it, but those that do can give to their ballets a power which is outside dance technique or even beauty. *The Rake's Progress* is not a "beautiful" work, nor has it great technical invention; but no one who sees it can doubt the quality of the mind that produced it.

Ballet's preoccupation for centuries with the fairy tale and the Greek myth, with its remoteness from modern psychology and life, was a drag on its powers of expression and imagination from which in some countries to-day, notably France, it has still not broken free. Æschylus, Sophocles and Euripides have, through poetry, raised the Greek heroic legend to a plane it is idle for ballet at this time to attempt to attain, especially since the Homeric ideals in conduct and religion have no practical significance for a contemporary democratic audience. The widening of subject matter through Fokine's revolt has opened up many new fields for the ballet composer, some of which Fokine himself never attempted to develop but which are to-day proving rich mining ground for the choreographer who has something interesting to say and the technical and mental equipment with which to say it.

Of what does this technical equipment consist? Ballet being created for performance in a theatre, the affinity of the choreographer to the dramatist is obvious, and like the poet who undertakes to write a play he must be governed by the theatre's laws and mould his material into dramatic form. Without this discipline, his creation will not become a living part of its new element; the pre-eminence of Shakespeare as a writer for the stage, in comparison with those many poets whose dramatic efforts withered into nothingness at first contact with the stage, rests above all things in this understanding of theatrical requirements. But if the choreographer must have a dramatist's skill in the presentation of characters and theme, his actual means of expression more approximate to those of the painter. Like the painter he must express his ideas through the medium of pictures, but in his case the difficulty of the task is intensified by the fact that each theme demands not one static picture merely but a series of moving pictures in which the form and beauty of composition are sustained in spite of the continual breaking up of the groups into action. The choreographer, in fact, must combine something of Leonardo da Vinci's sense of structure and balance in composition with Blake's power to express movement, of which a critic has written "vision is continuous and not instantaneous, and those, like Blake, who can make a figure run or swim or fly, always produce their effect by combining what happens at different instants of time." This continuity of vision is the essence of good choreography, and the relationship of pictures and figures to questions of time and space and aerial as well as horizontal perspective presents a problem which must equally be faced and mastered. No wonder, then, that Noverre urged choreographers to consult the creations of the most eminent painters, and through this study learn to avoid, as far as possible, that symmetry of figures which, by repetition, seems to present two separate pictures on one and the same canvas. It is this abnormal and lifeless symmetry in *ensemble*, as opposed to the true artist's sense of balance and visual rhythm in construction, that Fokine also later decries. "Nearer to Nature" is Noverre's demand,

and as long as artistic form is preserved and does not collapse, in the wrong hands, into constructional anarchy, it is a useful guide to the artist.

I have referred above to "visual rhythm." It is a necessary corollary, in ballet, of aural rhythm, and the expression through dance and movement of the music. Unless we can accept the theories of some modern American and German votaresses of the free dance, and of Serge Lifar, choreographer of the Paris Opera, in his *Ballet, Traditional to Modern*, that ballet can exist as a purely abstract art form without musical aid, the choreographer's task of creating pictures is governed by the necessity of also paralleling or reflecting the rhythm of the music. Critical assessment of ballet is based on a study of the homogeneity of its component parts—dance, theme, music and *décor*—and without music, or with a percussion accompaniment dictated by the choreographer, ballet tends to become reduced to the quite different medium of the dance recital. This is not progression but retrogression, a return to the primitive self-expression from which dance originally evolved, and it is perhaps significant that its advocates are those who have always based their dance creations primarily on their own individual talents as dancers. Certainly it is an easy way out for the unmusical dance composer; but such an anomaly should not exist and musicality is an essential in the really first-class choreographer.

How can this quality of musicality be defined? A choreographer or dancer can have a meticulous accuracy of metre without ever seeming really musical. A sense of rhythm, something far more instinctive and subtle in *nuance*, is essential, and a realisation of the *feeling* of the music more important than a painstaking reproduction of "beat." Stravinsky in his autobiography makes the interesting comment:"Choreographers are fond of cutting up a rhythmic episode of the music into fragments, of working up each fragment separately, and then striking the fragments together. By reason of this dissection, the choreographic line, which should coincide with that of the music, rarely does so." "Line" in dance, then, is melodic as well as visual, and its fluency must be preserved even when the choreography illustrates the harmony and counterpoint of the music. It is in the use of mass movement that the choreographer achieves the equivalent of orchestral "colour." Counterpoint, reduced to its simplest terms, is illustrated by the first entrance of Harlequin and Columbine in *Carnaval;* in Nijinsky's *Sacre du Printemps* it was revealed in the massed opposition of groups of dancers dancing lightly or heavily, in Helpmann's *Miracle in the*

Gorbals the two young lovers dance forestage in a lyrical counterpoint to the swaying lamentation of the crowd. Parallel with this sense of musical style and feeling there is, in the greatest choreographers, that touch of imagination, akin to poetry, which can illuminate a passage of the music with movement of unusual sensitiveness or dramatic relevance. The driving in of the crucifixion nails in *Dante Sonata* is such a moment, and Ashton's ballet throughout imaginatively translates the emotion and spirit of Liszt's Sonata into dramatic action.

Inventiveness in the use of dance technique is a necessary gift in the choreographer, though it should be realised that it is not the only or even always the predominant gift, and it exists in the beautiful and simple use of old steps as well as in the creation of new. The footwork in Fokine's most beautiful dance in *Carnaval* is based entirely on the simple little running steps of the *pas de bourrée*, the originality consisting in the patterns woven by the three dancers with their linked hands. An endless variety of effects of line can be achieved with the arabesque, and of architectural composition and flight with the "lift" of dancers in the air. And always the beauty and expressiveness of the dance will depend finally on the choreographer's use not only of the dancer's legs and feet but of the whole body. Steps alone are meaningless unless the line and rhythm and balance of the dance are continuous from foot to fingertips. The inventive powers of the choreographer can be gauged by the movements he creates for the arms and hands as well as for the feet. A study of the Miller's Dance in Massine's *Le Tricorne*, of the part of Duessa in Ashton's *The Quest* and the dances of the Attendant Spirit and river nymphs in Helpmann's *Comus* will emphasise this.

The choreographer's dependence on the dancer is obvious; the human body is both his tool and his material, the equivalent of the paint of the artist, the words of the poet, the marble or clay of the sculptor. There is, however, this difference, that whereas the creations of other artists (unless the painter has, like da Vinci, an unfortunate bent for scientific experiment with types of paint) remain as originally produced, those of the choreographer have no such permanency. The dramatist and composer are also dependent on the performer for the standard of their work in the theatre or concert hall, but in their case the written play and music score are available for study and comparison. The lack of a dance notation which will successfully record ballets for posterity makes such a check on the choreographer's intentions impossible, and his composition will in any case be governed to some extent by the capabilities of the dancers at his disposal.

It is in his masterly use of this human material, his adaptation of the lines and motions of the body and the dancers' style and personality to express the rôle, that the choreographer's craftsmanship can be judged. Frederick Ashton and Georges Balanchine both display this craftsmanship to a high degree, and both in creation mould their work directly on to the dancers. Some others—Nijinska, for instance, and de Valois—prefer to create their ballets mentally and on paper very fully before the first rehearsals, and to adapt their dancers, wherever possible, to these pre-conceived ideas. The first method tends to produce work in which the accent is on pictorial beauty and invention, the second ballets of character and ideas. Because of their rich use of the dancing material originally available the first are sometimes difficult to recast successfully, but provided that key phrase "to express the rôle" (i.e. not just to exploit the personal idiosyncrasies of the dancer) has been observed, and the work is of genuine quality, it may survive its original dancers even though their interpretation may not for some time be equalled. *Petrouchka* has outlasted Nijinsky just as *Hamlet* (the play) has outlasted a few great and many indifferent interpreters. It lives not because it was a vehicle for a great dancer, but because as a ballet it is an artistic whole and its tragedy directed by mind as well as movement.

I have mentioned the choreographer's dependence on the dancer for the fullest realisation of his ideas; what is less often stressed is the dancer's dependence on the choreographer. The dancer who lacks the opportunity to work under a good and creative choreographer is inevitably restricted in his artistic development; it is doubtful if even Karsavina would have become the complete and versatile artist she did if Fokine had not created for her a variety of parts which gave her full scope to widen her range of expression. The importance of high standards in choreography cannot therefore be overstressed; without them not only ballet itself but the art of the dancer degenerates. This is a lesson which must be absorbed if the new ballet companies continually being formed are to achieve any basis of artistic permanence.

CHAPTER III

SIMPLICITY AND THE CHOREOGRAPHER

THE rising popularity of ballet in war-time has been accompanied by an increase not only in the number of ballet companies, but also of practising choreographers. This is in some ways disturbing. It is obvious that under war-time conditions, with the inevitable drain on male personnel, the talent available is not sufficient to keep even one English ballet company at its pre-war level of achievement, let alone four or five, and if this is true of the dancing it is doubly true of the choreography.

It is worth remembering that over a period of twenty years the Diaghileff ballet produced only four choreographers of abiding importance—Fokine, Massine, Nijinska and Balanchine—and in the ten years following Diaghileff's death the Russian modern ballet repertoire, apart from some experimental works by the young Lichine and an occasional revival of Nijinsky's *L'Après Midi d'un Faune*, was still composed entirely of works by these four. The Sadler's Wells and Ballet Rambert companies between them have, during the fifteen years' serious existence of English ballet, produced hardly more choreographers of worth, though since these few are a generation younger than the Russians the choreographic outlook for English ballet is correspondingly more hopeful; the desertion of one of them to the Russian-American side not seriously altering the balance.

It is obvious, then, that talent for choreography is extremely rare, and since it involves so wide a basis of knowledge, not merely of dance movement and the dancer's physique, but also of art and music, it is not likely to be highly developed among the very young. Massine, an exception in producing some very good ballets while in the early twenties, was provided with unusual educational facilities by Diaghileff, which included study in the world's finest art galleries and museums; opportunities obviously outside the reach of the average young dancer of to-day. Fokine's genius also became apparent at an early age, but at the time of his first contact with Diaghileff and the production of his surviving ballets, starting with *Sylphides*, he was nearing thirty. So was Frederick Ashton when he left the Ballet Club and for the first time worked continuously with a major company, the Wells, on a larger stage.

Here, I think, we come to a point of outstanding significance: the immense value to the choreographer of experience on a small stage. It is natural for youth to want to spread its wings, to splash itself on to a large canvas; natural, but inadvisable, and the poorness of much of the choreography to be seen in England to-day is very frequently due to this cause, that a large stage and *corps de ballet* are available which the young and inexperienced choreographer is quite unable to use. Mastery of mass movement can only come from experience in the creation of pattern on a smaller scale, and it is lack of *pattern* in movement that is the most glaring fault of some of this work by young choreographers. The tendency is to overcrowd the stage, to over-elaborate, to choose too long a musical score and then fill up the ballet with irrelevancies, introducing dances for their own sake and thus holding up the progression and weakening the dramatic "bite" of the story. The basic lack is of that quality which every great choreographer possesses and, paradoxical though it may seem, never completely loses even in the handling of dancers "in the mass": the quality of simplicity.

Bernard Shaw has said that it took him half a lifetime to simplify his style to the requirements of good prose, and every writer will recognise the fundamental truth of this. At seventeen one spends endless time adding new long words to one's script; at thirty taking them out. Greatness always involves command of the simple as well as the complex, and it took great men to create the "Air on the G String" and the Sonnets as well as the Mass in B Minor and *Antony and Cleopatra*. This simplicity the great choreographers invariably possess, and it provides the basic pattern on which they embroider their richest effects. Immediately that pattern is lost mass movement becomes, not a ballet, but at best a pageant or spectacle, at worst a "scrum." Ashton's Ball Scene in *Apparitions* is a particularly fine example of a full company of dancers used in such a way that the pattern, though it flows and merges, is never lost, and at the same time the atmosphere of a dream is brilliantly sustained.

There have been great ballets based on a rich orchestration of movement, and "abstract" ballets usually fall into this category; but there have been great ballets, too, on a smaller scale, and the beauty of these usually rests in two things—simplicity and atmosphere. *Sylphides*, with its clear, flexible lines, is the obvious example; it is in fact a series of lovely, fluent groupings, each conveying the poetic atmosphere and occasionally pausing like a photographic "still," as in that beautiful arrangement of the *corps de ballet* in three groups like moonlit pools of water, a *coryphée* rising from the centre of each like a water lily. *Carnaval* and *Spectre de la Rose*, too, have essential simplicity, and like one of the more moving of English ballets, Antony Tudor's *Jardin Aux Lilas*, depend principally for their effect on a delicate evocation of atmosphere. The choreography in the Tudor ballet is, in fact, simple to the point of elementary, and the mood depends, as in *Spectre de la Rose*, very largely on the mimic quality of the dancers.

In character or narrative ballet, where more elaboration and the use of many dancers is involved, it is essential that all the movement on the stage should have character and meaning. Ninette de Valois has brilliantly achieved this in the first scenes of *The Prospect Before Us* and *The Rake's Progress* which, though filled with incidental detail, never seem to have redundancies, since every movement helps to build up character and contributes to one general impression. Incidentally it is, perhaps, here worth noting that in her early ballet *Création du Monde*, with a small company and very limited means, Miss de Valois achieved an impression of the creation of the earth which was more expressive, and remains in the memory far more vividly, than that created by Massine, with the full resources of Russian ballet and the Drury Lane stage, in *Seventh Symphony*. The writhing surge of plant-life in Miss de Valois's ballet was as graphic as the strokes of colour in a Van Gogh canvas, and the choreographer's brushwork had the same basis of simplicity and strength.

Robert Helpmann's *Hamlet* is an unusual example of simplicity of design which, on study, reveals itself as full of dramatic and psychological detail. Every gesture in this ballet has meaning, and the straight, flowing lines of the pattern sweep the action forward, and create pictures of beauty, with rare economy of means. Incidentally Helpmann is the first totally inexperienced choreographer to have been asked to create a ballet for the major English company, Sadler's Wells, but the choice in this case was justified since he was already a mature dancer of long experience with a good working knowledge of the company, a natural dramatic and musical instinct, and very definite standards of taste in painting and sculpture. Generally speaking, the refusal of the director, Ninette de Valois, to allow young and inexperienced artists, however promising, to cut their choreographic teeth at Sadler's Wells has been justified in the long run. There have been failures in the Wells repertoire, but they have been the failures of good choreographers (even the greatest produce some failures; Fokine produced many, especially in his later career) and not of fumbling immaturity. As a result the general level of achievement has been remarkably maintained.

Reports from America, in which country the main body of *emigré* (as distinct from Soviet) Russian talent has settled since the war, suggest that there the outlook is not so reassuring. With the dancing and choreographic talent shifting between several major companies America seems to have become a scene of feverish activity with, apart from Antony Tudor's steady residence as principal choreographer with the Ballet Theatre, disproportionately few permanent results. The failure of a further new company to obtain a public was significantly attributed in the American journal, *Dance News*, for December 1944 to its repertoire of "new ballets by choreographers not yet prepared to stage for a major ballet company."

It is here that England's good fortune in possessing a smaller-scale company of quality, the Ballet Rambert (formerly known as the Ballet Club), becomes apparent. Directed by Marie Rambert with the deliberate policy of encouraging young talent, and being therefore in a position to experiment without the loss of prestige that a larger company, expected to produce only mature and finished work, would suffer in the event of failure, this company, using a small stage, has provided young English choreographers with a practical and essential training in simplicity. It is, in fact, safe to say that both Antony Tudor in America and Frederick Ashton in England owe their ability to work successfully on a larger scale to their early encouragement by Madame Rambert and training with her company. The formation of a second company at Sadler's Wells will also provide training and opportunities that have been denied the inexperienced choreographer in the major Sadler's Wells company.

CHAPTER IV

BALLET AND THE PAINTER

IDEALLY considered, ballet represents the perfect fusion of music, design and dance, and the greatest ballets are those in which the work of composer, artist and choreographer is of the highest quality and in the most complete sympathy. All three creators are restricted by a common framework, the theme to be expressed, but the relationship between the choreographer and the composer and the choreographer and the artist has, in the conception of the ballet, a subtle difference.

The choreographer can, to a limited extent, indicate to the composer roughly what he requires at certain points in the action: a dramatic crescendo here, a waltz, a lyrical passage, there. He can also suggest a time limit for the scenes and variations. But since the entrance of the serious musician into ballet, this is the utmost extent of his influence, and if he is working to an existing score his subservience to the musician is complete, his only freedom being in the choice of appropriate music. In any case the nature of the choreography is determined by the rhythm of the music, and not a step can be devised until this is composed.

If the choreographer's creative impulse is disciplined by the music, that of the artist should, if the finest results are to be achieved, be governed to some extent by the form of the choreography. The easel artist conceives his pictures in terms of figures, grouping and background artistically correlated. Ballet is a series of pictures in motion, in which the lines and groupings created by the choreographer are constantly breaking, merging and re-forming. It is the artist's business to provide these pictures with a background which blends with their general flow and style, and costumes which allow freedom of movement, never obscure the dancing line, and of a colour scheme which remains effective in the changing positions of the dancers. There have been ballets in which costumes or scenery have so obscured the intention and detail of the choreography that one can only imagine they were designed purely on the basis of the scenario and without reference

19

to the type of choreography composed. Unless the artist works with, or after, the choreographer, there is always this danger.

The ballet artist, then, is not a free agent in the sense that the modern easel artist is free to express his genius, or sometimes merely his ego, in any manner he chooses. It is only the lesser artists, however, who lack the gift of compromise and adaptation. Musicians of the genius of Beethoven have deliberately created their finest work within the rigid framework of the sonata form, and the greatest painting of the Renaissance occurred under the dictation of patrons and in the form of church decoration of pre-arranged size and content. "The Last Supper" and Michelangelo's painting of the Sistine Chapel ceiling were both produced under these conditions. The freedom of the modern artist is, in any case, not absolute, the commercial dictatorship of the art dealer and buyer having replaced that of the patron.

Ballet can occupy for the modern artist the position held by the church for the artist of the Renaissance. Diaghileff might even be regarded as the modern successor to the mediæval patron, only a patron without restrictive impulses and with a wide artistic taste and flair. The scope of ballet as a medium is proved by the fact that some of the best work of artists such as Bakst, Benois, Picasso and Derain has been created for it, and it is significant that the title of the journal that preceded the richest creative period of Russian ballet was *The World of Art*.

Ballet, as an artistic force, has never been so strong as under Diaghileff's direction, and in England the easel, as opposed to the theatre, artist has remained fairly aloof. The standard of theatrical *décor* is increasingly high, and artists of the calibre of the late Rex Whistler and Oliver Messel, devoting their talents to the theatre and the ballet, have produced work which can compare with that of the Diaghileff artists. But a few swallows do not make a summer, and if the standard is to be maintained there must be a new influx of artists into the theatre, learning to adapt their gifts to its conditions and bringing to ballet the imaginative stimulus its very composition demands. The recent employment of easel artists such as John Piper, Graham Sutherland, Edward Burra and Leslie Hurry is therefore a good augury, however varying the initial success.

Ballet in one sense is an admirable medium for the easel painter. It is of necessity confined mainly to one level and if movement is not to be restricted there can be no question of rostrums, except in a limited degree; steps at the side of the stage, as in *Hamlet*, are almost

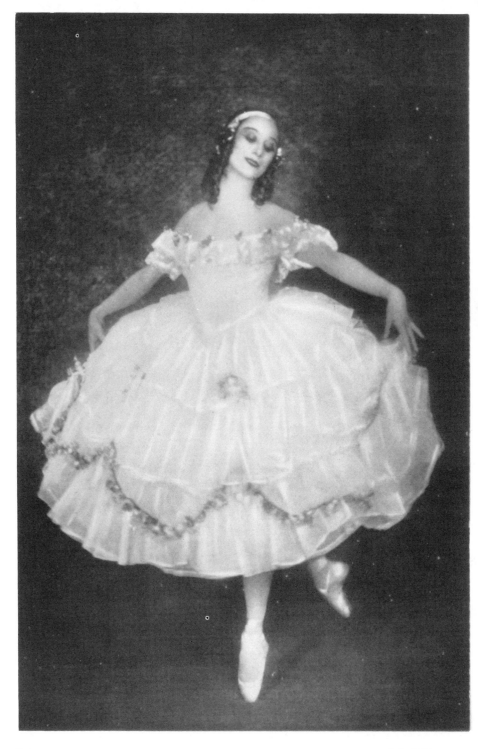

Anna Pavlova in *Christmas*

Plate II

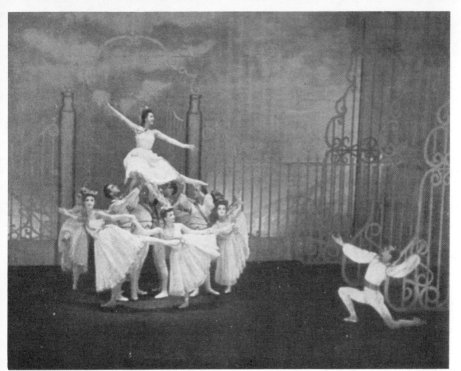

Plate III   (*Above*) Group and construction in Choreography
Les Rendezvous: Scene with Beryl Grey

Plate IV   (*Below*) Dancer in Variation
Alexis Rassine in *Les Rendezvous*

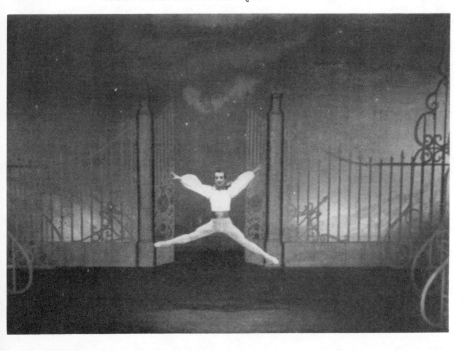

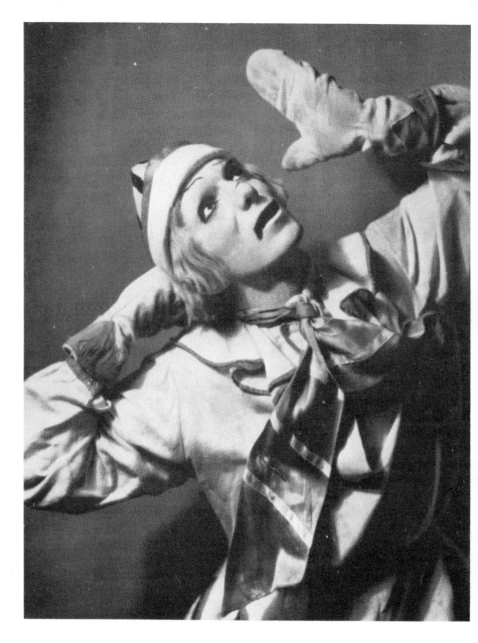

Russian Dance-Drama
Léonide Massine in *Petrouchka*

Plate V

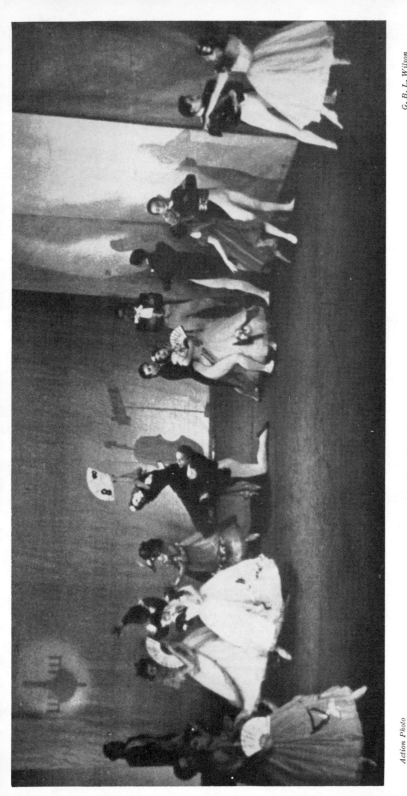

G. B. L. Wilson

The Ball Scene in *Apparitions*
Décor and costumes by Cecil Beaton

Plate VI

Plate VII

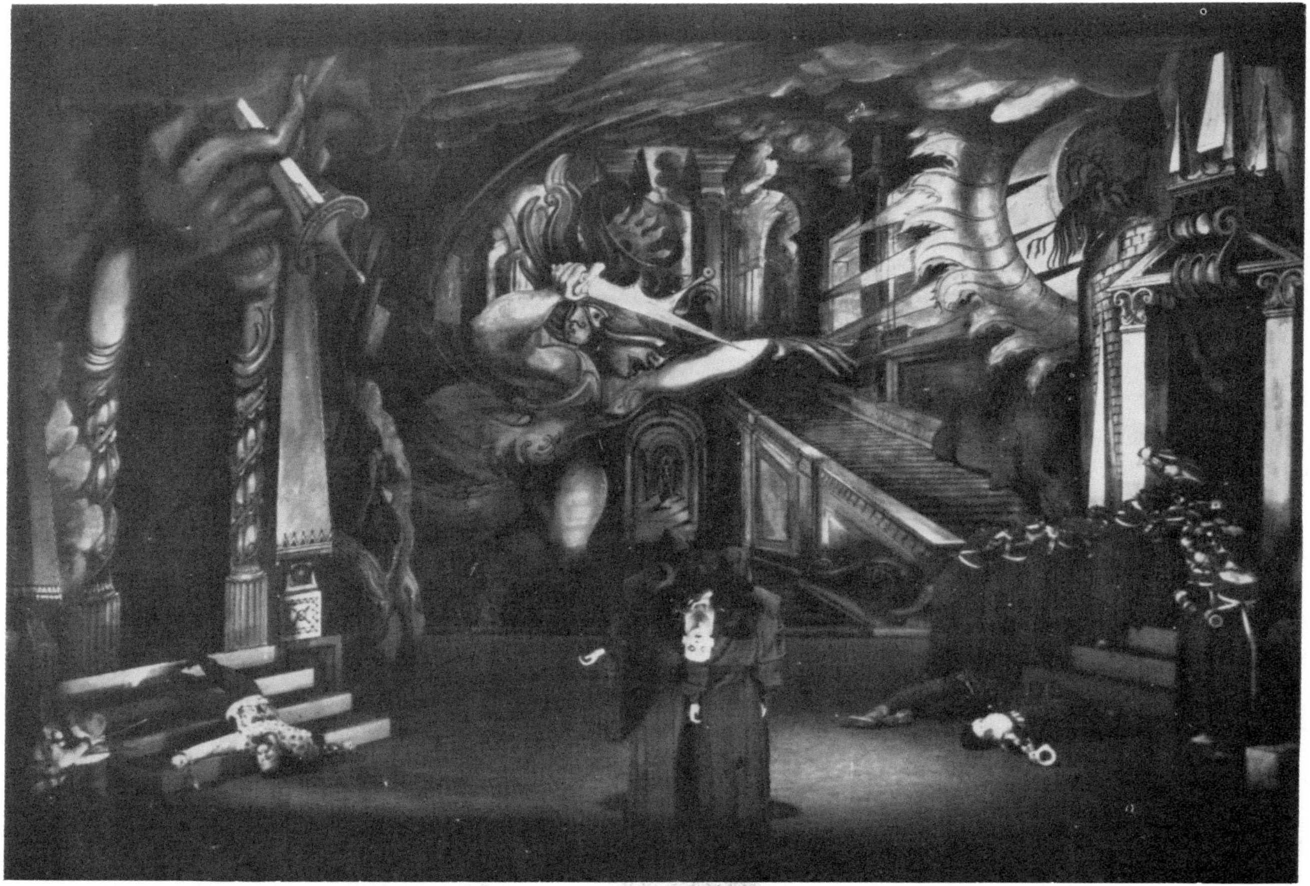

Shakespearean
Ballet: *Hamlet*

Opening and
final scene.

Décor by Leslie
Hurry.

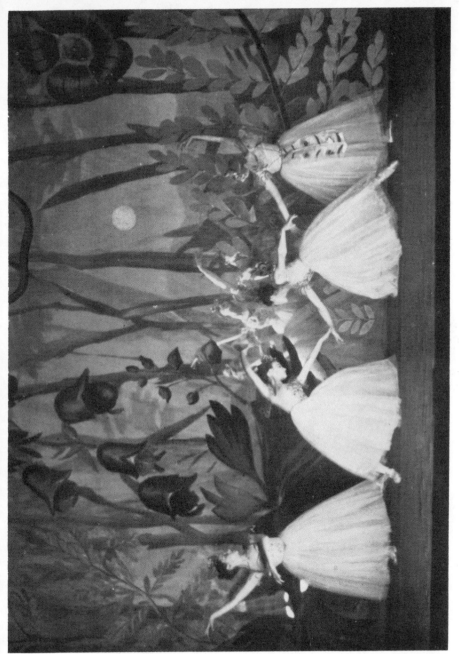

Evocation of the Romantic Period: Ballet in *A Midsummer Night's Dream*, Old Vic, 1937. *Décor* by Oliver Messel.

Plate VIII

Photo J. W. Debenham

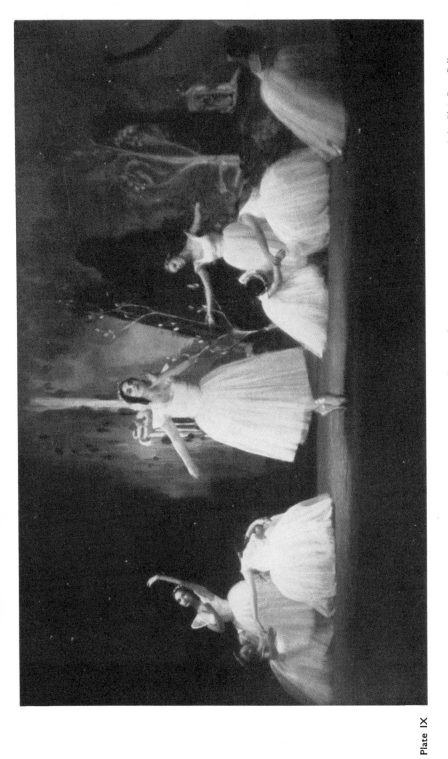

Plate IX

Les Sylphides: Pattern in the Prelude, Anne Ashley and the Ballet Rambert

Action Photo Peggy Delius

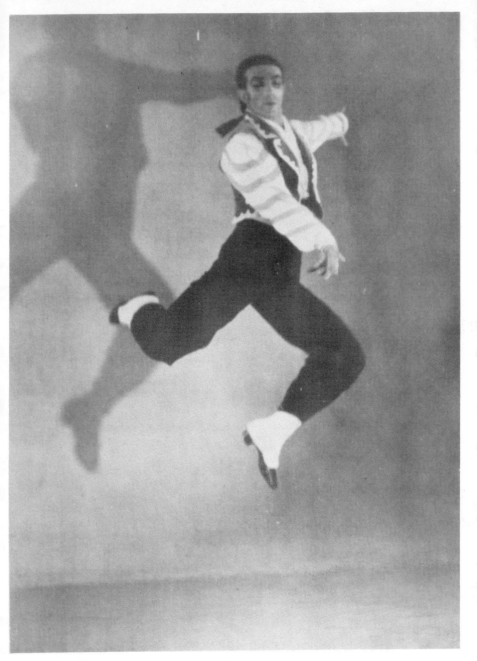

Le Tricorne
Miller's Dance: Léonide Massine

Plate X

the only means of creating another plane for effects of grouping and still allowing the groups to dissolve and the dancers move without a break to another part of the stage. The *décor* is therefore concentrated in the backcloth, which becomes an enlarged canvas for the artist. The fine architectural draughtsmanship of a Rex Whistler can be employed here with infinite variety. Landscape can be purely pastoral, as in *Comus*, romantically conceived, as in Benois's *Sylphides* with its ruined chapel, or atmospheric as in Roerich's *Prince Igor*, which is like no scene on earth, but, with its barren outlines drenched in a blood-red, scorching sunset (or perhaps the reflected fires of the Polvotsian camp), magnificently reflects the barbaric splendour and virility of the Fokine dances. The "abstract" ballet provides for limitless imaginative range, but it is most important of all, perhaps, here that the artist has a sensitive feeling for choreographic line. The finest "abstract" ballet *décor* is that of Sophie Fedorovitch in *Dante Sonata;* the plain black backcloth, with its few wavering white lines and parallel strokes, is classically simple and seems subtly to follow the flow of the dancing. The rest is achieved by lighting, an important accessory on which the designer is (sometimes unfortunately) dependent. It adds enormously, for instance, to the work of the surréalist, the painter of dreams, whose effectiveness as an artist for ballet has been apparent in *Jeux d'Enfants* and *Hamlet*. Ballet has small use for what might be called pedestrian surréalism, the mere painting in juxtaposition of unrelated objects; but the surréalist of imagination, whose images have a common significance all tending to create one atmosphere or effect, is another matter. Leslie Hurry's *Hamlet*, with its coherence, power and superb sense of colour, fulfils these conditions and his *décor* must rank as one of the greatest in the history of ballet.

Ballet is by its nature unrealistic, a stylised convention, and the Impressionist school of painting, with its absence of form and concentration on effects of light, its attempt to put into paint things exactly as they strike the vision of the artist in an instant of time, would probably have been of little use to it. In view of the dancer's inherent inability to turn himself into a cube, it is surprising that the work of a Cubist such as Picasso should be so effective. That the figures have not seemed odd against the Cubist *décor* must be in some measure due to the costume design. Costume in ballet must of necessity rely on *impression* rather than accuracy; the dancer's limbs must be unhampered, and if the designer can suggest the period as well so much

the better. Oliver Messel's design for the Lady in *Comus* is ideal in
this respect. A sense of colour, not only with regard to pictorial
beauty, but also to character and dramatic effect, is essential. The black
and white scheme of *Dante Sonata* dramatically realises the significance
of the theme, and the single figure of Comus in red, a pivotal flame
around which the other characters revolve like moths, is æsthetically
dead right. Colour in ballet can blaze, but it must also blend. Bakst's
riot of colours in *Scheherazade* never scream at each other; those in
Jardin Public did, and one could only echo Gilbert's Lady Jane: "Red
and yellow! Primary colours! Oh, South Kensington!" The most
striking effects can be achieved against the plainest background, as
Cecil Beaton realised in *Apparitions*, where the simplicity of the *décor*
accentuates the rainbow radiance of the ball dresses and the vivid
violet and red of the monks. The pastel background of Beaton's
ball scene, with its shadowed symbols of an orchestra, is a fine example
of suggestion in ballet *décor*.

Suggestion being a corollary of fantasy, it is interesting to find the
surréalist Leslie Hurry chosen as designer for a new production of
Lac des Cygnes for Sadler's Wells. There is a school of thought that
maintains that spectacular magnificence in the Maryinsky manner is
essential to the classical ballets, but it is worth remembering it was
against Maryinsky Theatre standards that the Diaghileff artists revolted.
These ballets have survived in the world repertoires not as spectacles
but as supreme examples of classical technique, and the revelation of
the dancing line is the first and only essential rule for the designer.
I suggest that Diaghileff's production of *The Sleeping Princess* failed
partly for this reason, that it overloaded the ballet with finery which
obscured at times the choreographic line (a subsequent complaint by
one of the principal dancers that the costumes were too heavy to
dance in bears out this impression). The tendency in recent years has
been to simplify the dancer's silhouette and strip away all unnecessary
trimmings, and Nijinsky in a photograph from *Le Pavilion d'Armide*,
once considered the last word in ballet design, strikes us now as
fantastically over-dressed. This is all to the good. The ideal, perhaps,
for classical *décor* would be the structural proportion and harmony
of the Greeks, and draughtsmanship is essential. The vision scene in
the original Wells production of *The Sleeping Princess* failed because
the modern style of the backcloth suggested bad drawing totally out
of keeping with the classical choreography, and the dresses of the
corps de ballet were fussy and ugly in line. Hurry in his *décor* and

costumes for *Lac des Cygnes* has not made this mistake; although his emphasis is on romantic fantasy and he does not attempt a Grecian classicism, the line of the dance is not obscured, his costumes are light and easy to wear and he achieves spectacle without sacrifice of draughtsmanship.

Ballet provides a third dimension to the painter, and it would be interesting to see the work of sculptors, such as Epstein and Henry Moore, in this medium. No dancer is ever going to look like a figure by Moore (one hopes), but Moore deals in symbols of life, and symbolism is a legitimate element in ballet *décor*. Among painters those with linear strength and balance are more likely to be successful in stage work than those whose draughtmanship is less definitive in outline; Edward Burra, with his boldness of colour and contour and macabre sense of the masque, might be successful in types of ballet quite different to the slum realism of his *Miracle in the Gorbals*, and Paul Nash and Matthew Smith, representing symbolic imagination and colour respectively, are artists who might bring much of value to ballet. The choreographer is an artist whose work is incomplete without the finishing touch of the painter; the greater the choreographer, the greater the painter he deserves. The reverse also applies. No *décor* survives a bad ballet, and if great artists are to be attracted to the medium they must be given something worth working on. Cocteau said that all art is decorative that is not felt, and if artists are to produce something more than mere decoration ballet must be something more than "dancing for dancing's sake"; it must be a work of art the artist can feel. Which brings us back, as always, to Noverre.

CHAPTER V

SHAKESPEAREAN BALLET

THERE are now two ballets based on plays by Shakespeare in the repertoire of English Ballet companies; Soviet Russia has produced two others, *The Merry Wives of Windsor* and *Romeo and Juliet;* and a fifth, also based on *Romeo and Juliet*, has been created by the English choreographer Antony Tudor in New York.

There is no doubt that the trend of ballet lately has been away from the "abstract" and mainly technical and towards the "literary"; the work of the younger choreographers—David Lichine, Tudor, Helpmann—has all shown this tendency, though coloured in each case by individuality of style and the psychological impression of their generation. In the English ballet, partly owing to a rich literary heritage, the theatre traditions of the masque and pantomime, and the natural English gift for characterisation, the trend is particularly marked. *The Rake's Progress*, the most "English" ballet yet created and a masterpiece of its kind, is bound to have its influence on the future, and the criticism which would discourage dramatic ballet as suchis, in fact, discouraging the development of English Ballet with a style and idiom of its own.

It was inevitable, in these circumstances, that English choreographers would turn to Shakespeare as well as to Milton, Spenser and the Bible (which it has always been a charming national characteristic to regard as a purely British concern) for inspiration. There is no reason why this should be considered artistically illegitimate. Artists have always drawn on each other for subject matter, and few of the greatest works of art, outside music, are pure invention. The Greek dramatists drew on local mythology, just as Shelley, T. S. Eliot and Eugene O'Neill have drawn on the Greeks; not a story of Shakespeare's was his own; the legends of Faust and Orpheus and the stories of the Bible have inspired poets, painters and musicians in every country and period. Ballet is a form of illustration, and the translation of *Hamlet* into balletic terms is no more invalid, in itself, than Blake's illustrations to the Book of Job or Verdi's musical interpretation of *Othello* and *Falstaff*, two works which represent the finest artistic achievement of Italian opera and their composer. The artistic value of the translation depends only on the degree of creative imagination possessed by the artist, and his ability to give to the original a new significance in his own medium.

It is obvious that artists of this calibre are rare; to one Verdi there will be a dozen Ambroise Thomases, and to one Blake a dozen Holman Hunts. In ballet it is only the choreographer who is a master of his medium, who has an innate sympathy with and understanding of his author, and something original of his own to express, who will be successful.

The English ballets of *Twelfth Night* (produced by the International Company) and *Hamlet* are, judged by these criteria, illuminating examples of failure and success in Shakespearean Ballet.

Twelfth Night fails in part because of a fundamental defect of planning, and in part because the choreography nowhere reflects the poetic genius or richness of character of the original. Unimaginatively following the play's sequence of events, the ballet never becomes more than a pale copy or develops an entity of its own. Scenes such as the duel of Viola and Aguecheek and Feste's "Sir Topaz" impersonation—with its repetition intact of the clumsy traditional "business" with the stilts—are no more balletic than the average stage production of the play. Of the characters only Maria, Feste and Aguecheek are even adequately translated; Sir Toby is a blank, Malvolio a mere figure of farce, Viola's exquisite qualities of poetry and despriz'd love, of sunshine shot with tears, never suggested. Andrée Howard has arranged one or two charming dances, but she is hampered throughout by the plan of the production (which was not her own). At one moment only the ballet points the direction that Shakespearean Ballet, if it is to produce anything of value, must take. Orsino's dream-dance with Olivia and her ladies, set oddly enough to the "Death of Åse" from *Peer Gynt*, is a purely imaginative suggestion of Orsino's longing for Olivia and her elusiveness, as well as being choreography of beauty in mood and pattern.

It is significant that Robert Helpmann's *Hamlet* is planned through-out on this imaginative basis. By taking as his cue "And in that sleep of death what dreams may come," and building the entire ballet on the fevered and distorted memories of the dying Hamlet, Helpmann has given himself absolute freedom in which to create a purely balletic vision of the theme, a work which has original genius as a ballet as well as being vividly suggestive of the play's psychological and emotional content. It is, in fact, a critical *commentary* on Shakespeare's play and as such something quite new in ballet. A well-known Shakespearean producer has said to me that Helpmann has, in his opinion, by a stroke of genius found "the only possible way" of expressing the play in ballet terms, and of the ten or twelve productions of *Hamlet* I have personally seen not more than three or four have conveyed the spiritual essence of the play as forcefully as Helpmann has done in this twenty-minute ballet. This is in part due to the fact that Helpmann himself is a born Hamlet (he has since played the part with success in the theatre); but only in part.

It is true that the subtlety of detail with which Helpmann has illustrated his theme must be lost on those onlookers without a fairly thorough knowledge of the play, but it is not true, in my opinion, that the audience without this knowledge is bewildered by the ballet. The dramatic essentials of character and theme are sharply defined, and their impact on the audience obvious at every performance. It is this imagination in detail which has helped to build a vital and exciting whole, and the audience is subconsciously aware of this even though its richness and significance—as in the case of all great ballets—can only be fully appreciated after the ballet has been seen a number of times.

The suggestion has been made that *Hamlet*, in view of its choreographic style, is not truly a ballet. The dance in *Hamlet* is, in fact, an individual development of the ideals of Noverre and Fokine, that sought to replace brilliance of footwork and conventional gesture by expressiveness of the whole body, to make ballet, in Noverre's words, "speak to the soul through the eyes." Fokine dispensed with stylised mime, but in *Scheherazade* mime and dance are still fairly distinct elements. In *Hamlet* the logical progression has been reached and the dividing line between mime and dance has disappeared. *Hamlet* is no more a mimed play than *The Green Table* or *Dante Sonata;* all three are ballets which could only be performed by trained dancers who can express themselves emotionally as well as technically.

In all living art there is an element of change, and if ballet is to remain a vital force it must allow its creators more than one mode of expression. English Ballet has developed with such rapidity and variety just because it has been fortunate enough to possess three choreographers of such marked difference of style as Frederick

Ashton, Ninette de Valois and Robert Helpmann. There is room for all kinds of ballet—technical, "abstract," dramatic, Shakespearean; the only essential is the genuine creative imagination and integrity of the choreographer. If he possesses these qualities his work cannot but enrich the art he serves.

CHAPTER VI

THE CLASSICAL BACKGROUND

UP to the present this book has dealt with the art of the ballet as that art has been understood since the time of Fokine: a unity in which dance, drama, music and design are intimately correlated, and the whole created not for spectacular or acrobatic but for expressive purposes. Yet in the repertoire of all important ballet companies some ballets remain from the pre-Fokine era, a recognised and necessary foundation of dance technique and style in the purest form, and the medium through which the standard of execution of the highest form of classical dancer, the ballerina or *danseur noble*, must still be judged.

When, in the early nineteenth century, the female dancer first rose upon the tips of her toes, instead of the half or three-quarter point which, in a soft ballet shoe, was the most she had previously attained, what is now known as the "classical" ballet received its first impetus, and an emphasis on sheer visual beauty and technical prowess began to be developed. Coinciding with the romantic movement in poetry, painting and music, dancing on full point came at just the right moment as a means to suggest the poetry of flight, and thus give the finishing touch of spirituality to the heroine of the tales of sprites and sylphs which for some years to come were to dominate ballet in the theatre. The romantic element was reinforced moreover by the emergence about this time of Taglioni, whose ethereality and extraordinary elevation made her peculiarly fitted for the expression of that romantic Byronic impulse, the conflict of the flesh and the spirit, which now entered and permeated ballet alongside the other arts. *La Sylphide*, created for Taglioni by her father, was the most famous product of the period, and though it has not survived, its spirit lives to-day in the purely abstract dances of *Les Sylphides*, created by Fokine as an evocation of the Romantic era and named by him in memory of the story-ballet in which the great dancer of the past made her principal triumph. The popular Romantic mechanism of flying fairies has rarely been revived in the ballet theatre, though it was introduced by Ninette de Valois with charming grace into her incidental ballets, to Mendelssohn's music, in the Old Vic Romantic-period production of *A Midsummer Night's Dream* in 1937.

Yet the concentration of Romantic ballet was not entirely on the "fey." The French Revolution and the writings of Rousseau had infused into artists a new awareness of the spirit of democracy and the life of the peasant and common people, and this influence too began to be felt in ballet. The heroes of Greek mythology, formerly the main source of ballet characterisation, disappeared; the sylphs and naïads fell in love with mortals of humble origin and played out their tragedy among the natural scenes of country life. Folk dance entered ballet side by side with the classical, and the contrast of earthly passion with the faëry was emphasised by the dancing of Taglioni's "opposite," the opulent and vital Fanny Elssler. The human and spiritual qualities meet in one character in *Giselle*, the one ballet of the period to survive, and the ballerina has thus added to her heritage the greatest and most emotionally varied of all her parts, the peasant girl who, finding her lover to be of noble birth and, as she believes, her betrayer, goes mad, kills herself with his sword, and later returns, a spirit, to save him from death at the hands of the Wilis, fatal and seductive sprites of German mythology. The part is one that requires an actress and dancer of the highest order, one who can combine human qualities of warmth and gaiety, suffering and distraction, with an intangible lightness that in the second scene becomes pure spirit. The dance arrangement of the leading part and the *corps de ballet* is a perfect example of French romantic classicism, the second Act *pas de deux* being an expression of emotion through pure dance, a love duet of delicate suggestion, and the choreography and grouping throughout having considerable beauty of line, pattern and invention. The choreographer was Coralli, helped it is generally believed by Jules Perrot, who with the shifting of the main ballet scene from Paris to St. Petersburg staged the ballet in Russia, where it was later revised slightly by Petipa. It is in this form, varied little in spirit from the original production of 1841, that *Giselle* has returned to Europe in our own time, the ballet in which Pavlova, Spessivitseva and our own Markova and Margot Fonteyn have achieved their highest distinction as dancers and expressive artists.

The music of Adolph Adam to *Giselle*, though not of the first quality, is tuneful, dramatically appropriate, and of higher standard than that usually created for ballet in this period, and it was a pupil of his, Délibes, who many years later composed the music for the only other French ballet of last century which survives in world repertoires to-day. This was *Coppélia*, produced in Paris in 1870, the year of the Prussian invasion, and a gay and brilliant vehicle for classical dancing which has outlasted the degenerate ballets of its period mainly because of its sparkling and well-orchestrated score and piquant light comedy "doll" story.

The seeds of the French ballet's artistic disintegration were already apparent in Gautier's writings when the art was in its most flourishing condition. Adulation of the dancer outweighs all other considerations, and the subject matter is becoming stereotyped. "Dancing," wrote Gautier, "consists of nothing more than the art of displaying beautiful shapes in graceful positions and the development from them of lines agreeable to the eye; it is mute rhythm, music that is seen. Dancing is little adapted to render metaphysical themes; it only expresses the passions; love, desire, with all its attendant coquetry; the male who attacks and the female who feebly defends herself is the basis of all primitive dances." It is easy to see how under this philosophy ballet may become in time a mere exhibition of sentimental coquettishness, and result in the artistic puerilities of Edwardian ballet at the French Opera and in the English music hall.

The pure—as opposed to romantic—classical ballet which grew up during the same period in Russia had a similar concentration on the "art of displaying beautiful shapes" and on the executive brilliance of the dancer, and far less interest in dramatic expression than French romantic ballet in its highest achievement, *Giselle*. But that "art of displaying beautiful shapes" it brought to a high degree of formalised loveliness, and the dying out of great dancers in France was accompanied by a corresponding emergence of fine Russian dancers trained in the State Academy founded originally by the Empress Anne in 1735. Under Marius Petipa, a French choreographer who came to Russia in 1847 and remained throughout the century, Russian ballet developed technique to a perfection which owed its final polish to the infusion of technical prowess learned from visiting Italian dancers of the Milan Academy, where Carlo Blasis's system of training was still followed. "The secret of the development of Russian dancing," wrote the dancer and teacher Nicholas Legat, "lay in the fact that we learnt from everybody and adapted what we learnt to ourselves. We copied, borrowed from, and emulated every source that gave us inspiration, and then, working on our acquired knowledge and lending it the stamp of the Russian national genius, we moulded it into the eclectic art of the Russian ballet."

Only three of Petipa's vast output of ballets survive in England: *Lac des Cygnes, The Sleeping Beauty* and *Casse Noisette*. They survive probably because alone of Petipa's ballets the music, by Tchaikovsky, is of a quality that far transcends that of the others. It was a period in which the work of the ballet musician and designer was of indifferent value by concert or easel standards, and both were in complete subservience to the choreographer. Ballet was the art of the Court, under the patronage of the Czar and attended mainly by the aristocracy, and the human element hardly entered into it. Its theme was the spectacular fairy tale, and lavishness its key. But in these ballets by Tchaikovsky it is possible to see choreographic construction of faultless pattern and purity of "line," and solo dancing which exploits the most brilliant resources of classic technique with nobility of style in the dancer. The dancer's body becomes an instrument of physical beauty in which the line flows unbroken from foot to fingertips, and poise and balance attain dignity through perfect control. Nor is the dance necessarily abstract or unemotional. The peak of the ballet, the *Adagio*, is at its best a love duet of dramatic and nerve-tingling excitement, and in the second Act of *Lac des Cygnes*, reputedly by Petipa's assistant Ivanov, it becomes, if properly danced, a lyric expression of a love tender, "fey" and doomed. Much of *Lac de Cygnes* has, in fact, in contrast to Petipa's glittering third Act, a poetic romanticism of design that almost anticipates Fokine, and it is an interesting fact that, many years before Duncan's attempt to express great music through dance had influenced Fokine in his ballet reforms, Ivanov was producing ballets to the music of Beethoven and similar composers.

Of Petipa himself Legat writes that his principal attention was "to grace and beauty of line and pose." The rot set in, as it always will when an art ceases to have contact with human life, and becomes purely spectacular and technical (concentration on "toe" dancing became, in particular, excessive); but the visual beauty of Russian classical ballet at its best is based on a clarity of grouping and aristocracy of movement that should be preserved, and give some meaning to the designation "classic" when its formal simplicity of line is compared to that of classic Greek architecture. It is interesting to remember, too, that the derivative of the word "classic" in art is the

Roman "classici," denoting the highest class of property owner as opposed to the lowest, the "proletarii." Since the term "classical" cannot, in ballet as in other arts, apply to the Grecian—for of Greek dance we know nothing beyond what can be reconstructed from bas reliefs and vases—it is perhaps appropriate that the period of ballet's highest development in the atmosphere of the Court should have become identified with the patrician epithet "classical."

The classic technique is the vocabulary of ballet, a vocabulary evolved in the theatre, via the Court ballroom, from the spontaneous steps of peasant dances. It is a highly developed, refined and stylised basis with many points of departure, and into which new elements from all kinds of dance are constantly being infused by the choreographer. As a result in England to-day *Lac des Cygnes* may be performed in the same repertoire with a ballet like *The Wise Virgins*, in which the hand movements are derivative from Hindu dances, and *Dante Sonata*, in which barefoot dancing inspired by the Central European style is performed with the requisite suppleness by classically-trained dancers. Yet the basic foundation is not dispensed with, any more than the musician and the writer dispense with the accepted groundwork of notation, grammar and language, however they may evolve new forms within the old vocabularies. When a writer, James Joyce, attempts this his work passes outside the comprehension—or averred comprehension—of all but the exclusive intellectual *coterie;* it loses its contact with the people. When a dancer—in the words of the American enthusiast and critic of the free dance, John Martin—attempts "the creation of movement directly out of experience without resort to vocabulary," she is faced with a vacuum a lifetime cannot expect to fill, and the dance becomes concentrated, far more than in classical ballet, on the personal self-expression of one individual.

A big enough mind, such as that of Kurt Jooss, will grasp this soon enough, and attempt to merge some of the discoveries of classic technique with those of the newer school of movement (though as a result he will almost certainly, like Jooss at the International Congress of the Dance which he organised at Essen, be rended by both sides as a desecrator). But when Mary Wigman, sensing something the same need for a solid foundation, makes as she thinks the profound discovery that "without form there is no dance," and Martin writes that with Wigman dance "touches for the first time in many centuries its common ground with theatre," one remembers Beaujoyeux's identification of ballet, three and a half centuries ago, with the Archimedes principles of geometrical proportions, and its development by Noverre and Fokine as an art governed by the laws of drama and the theatre; and one wonders at the *naïveté* of those who were born yesterday.

CHAPTER VII

THE VALUE OF CLASSICAL MIME

IN performances of *Lac des Cygnes* by the de Basil, Russian-American and some English companies it has been customary for the Diaghileff shortened version of this ballet to be used, in which a good but dramatically quite meaningless dance sequence is substituted for the traditional passage of mime between the Prince and Swan Princess. This practice gives rise to the question of whether stylised mime is worth preserving either for its own sake or in the education of dancers and choreographers.

There is a disturbing and frequently expressed opinion among balletgoers that classical mime is to-day valueless and outmoded as a means of expression, and as eminent a critic as Arnold Haskell has written that "in *Swan Lake* mime remains as a rather tedious interruption of the dance; so much so that in many versions it has been heavily curtailed, and with no loss." The Sadler's Wells Ballet Company, on the other hand, has always included the full mime passages in its performance of classical works and the teaching of mime in the syllabus of its school, and the opinion of the Sadler's Wells director as to the value of this is shared by a number of dancers.

The criticism of classical mime seems to fall under two headings: (*a*) it is meaningless to a modern audience not initiated into the significance of the sign language, and (*b*) since Fokine's rejection of stylised gesture, his demand that the dancer shall be expressive not only with his hands but with every part of his body, and his revolutionary conception of ballet as a fluid whole in which the mime is expressed through the dance or newly-created gesture, conventional mime as a separate entity is no longer artistically permissible. The last criticism, superficially a truism, proceeds actually from a confusion of two separate issues. No one will deny that ballet has progressed artistically beyond the point where classical mime-gesture can be used by a modern choreographer as a link between dance episodes, except possibly with a humorous "period" twist as Fokine has done with

34

Pierrot, Harlequin and Columbine in *Carnaval;* but *Lac des Cygnes, The Sleeping Beauty, Coppélia* and the first Act of *Giselle* were built in this period style and to attempt to alter their fundamental construction is to destroy either the dramatic progression of their story or the beauty and completeness of their dance arrangement, which still sets a standard in classical line and technique. Take out the mime scene from *Lac des Cygnes,* Act II, and this dance standard is still maintained; but the meaning of the dancing and the story it illustrates, which is still apparent when the mime is retained, is obscured and the one-Act version becomes nothing more than a *suite de danses.* There is a further interesting point which might be considered: the relationship of the music to the mime and dance. A distinguished conductor and musician has, in fact, expressed the view that Tchaikovsky's music for the mime passages is of a different style to that composed for the dance episodes, an "accompaniment" to the gestures, and no dance substituted for these scenes is musically satisfying for this reason.

The assertion that the classical sign language is difficult to understand is not borne out by the facts. There are no textbooks in which classical ballet mime may be studied, but it is obvious from the reactions of the modern audience, particularly in the humorous episodes of *Coppélia* if these are well done, that the general import of the gestures has been fully grasped. The gestures needing explanation are small in number; that for "mother," for instance, the hands crossed lightly upon the breast, is not readily clear, though once its meaning is known it is possible to appreciate the expressive resignation of the gesture. The gestures jar only when the scene in any case borders on the melodramatic; Hilarion in *Giselle* is a part notoriously difficult to mime convincingly and 'Giselle's rejection of him seems overemphatic. But the mime-gesture for "dancing," hands wreathed gaily and lightly above the head, is particularly effective in this ballet in suggesting Giselle's fatal passion for the dance, and the dramatic finality of the "death" gesture, hands descending *à bas* with the wrists crossed, has here a tragic significance. In comedy vein many will have been amused by Dr. Coppelius's denial to the still-suspicious Franz—fingers pointing up from the head like small devil's horns—of his villainous intentions, and by that charming little passage in *The Sleeping Beauty* when the King says in effect to his daughter, "You're quite grown-up now, and old enough to be married. Here are four young princes willing to take on the job . . . "

It is in *Lac des Cygnes,* however, that the beauty and expressiveness of classical mime is most effectively conveyed, and all the mime passages have a genuine romantic feeling. The serenity and grace of the gesture to denote a person's beauty, with its lovely sweeping movement of the hand clockwise around the face, the old tutor's reluctance to go hunting, the Prince's negation, hands lightly crossed and uncrossed, of his desire to marry or intention to hurt the fearful Swan Princess, her narration of her enchantment and possible release, poised tip-toe like a bird winged for flight, the moving little passage in the last act when two of the swans, with a grave lifting of the hands, try to raise the spirits of their Queen, and the later one in which the Prince, too, vainly tries to dissuade her from taking her life: these fragments of mime keep the drama constantly alive, and the characters moving and real even in this atmosphere of the fairy tale. They are, of course, not easy to perform well and for their full expressiveness demand absolute sincerity, intelligence and clear-cut but fluent gesture from the dancers. Some of the best mimes have found that it gives their mime greater conviction if they silently speak the dialogue to themselves while making the gestures. Phrasing is essential; it is difficult to grasp the meaning of a sentence if the words are spoken disjointedly, and mime also depends for its meaning on the "words" flowing smoothly and being phrased together to make a coherent "sentence." Equal expressiveness and response between the two "speakers," in a scene such as that between Odette and Siegfried in Act II of *Lac des Cygnes*, is also necessary, and the mime of Margot Fonteyn and Robert Helpmann in this scene is a pattern in this respect. No two other dancers in my memory have mimed it with such mutual sympathy and lucidity. Their comedy scenes together in *Coppélia* are also notable for their intuitive timing and response. A comparison of any two productions of *Coppélia* will show how this old-fashioned type of comedy mime varies in spontaneity and humour with the dancers.

These gestures of classical mime are expressive because they are fundamentally based on the natural movements and reactions of normal life. Some of them may have survived from the mime of ancient Greece and their effectiveness has been tried and proved over a number of centuries. Mimed gesture of some kind appears in the folk dance of every country and even the dances of the East. The Indian poet Tagore wrote of Balinese dancing: "The tongue is silent, but the whole body does the talking by signs as well as by movements." Joan Lawson, the critic and dancer, in her lecture-recitals to the Forces performs a Circassian folk dance, probably centuries old, in which the phrases "I love you" and "Will you marry me?" occur in the identical sign language of classical ballet mime.

Those choreographers who completely throw away this store of gesture accumulated from the past are sometimes limiting their powers of expression more than they realise. It may explain why some of the movement of the Ballets Jooss, in spite of the claims made for it, is actually curiously inexpressive, and when in *Company at the Manor* the women servants rush on to the stage shaking their fists above their heads little is conveyed except indignation, although apparently they are supposed to have related to the butler the full story of the scandalous change-over of the pairs of lovers. The choreographer trained in classical mime can, on the other hand, and without ever departing from Fokine's principle of the artistic merging of mime and dance, freely adapt that mime into his work with considerable gain to its dramatic meaning. The tragic and expressive dance of the Girl in *The Rake's Progress* has woven into it the same beautiful gesture, hands descending from the eyes, with which the Swan Princess tells of her mother's tears. Ninette de Valois has similarly in *Job* taken the simplest of mime gestures, the outflung arm and pointing finger, and given it a new significance by a wheeling overhead movement of sweeping malevolence. It occurs when Satan, from the throne of God, marks out Job as his prey. Even when the movement in a ballet is not obviously derived from classical mime, a knowledge of and training in that mime helps to give the choreographer an intuitive feeling for expressive gesture. Ashton's first scene in *The Quest* contains examples of gesture which, although freshly imagined, have the simplicity and expressiveness of pure classical mime, and the tranquil beauty and breadth of Helpmann's gestures as the Stranger in *Miracle in the Gorbals* are of the same genre.

Arnold Haskell has said that the classics are the grammar and syntax of the ballet, and if this is true of the dance it is also true of the mime. This, too, plays a valuable part in the forming of expressive artists: the dancer who can mime well in classical ballet will usually prove the most expressive interpreter of modern works, and the choreographer who is able to draw on the rich material of the past is the one most likely to produce progressive and lasting work. Voltaire's "Every present event is born of the past, and is father of the future" may be applied to art as well as to politics.

CHAPTER VIII

THE DANCER AS AN ARTIST

NOVERRE in 1760 published his *Lettres sur la Danse* with one principal aim: to demonstrate the difference between mechanical technique and that genius which places dancing beside the imitative arts. It was a plea for dancers "to combine ideas with the graces of their bodies," a protest both against the dancers' tendency to become "beautiful machines" and the audience's demand merely "to be shown the difficulties of the art."

The whole history of dancing since has been a constant pull between these two conceptions of the dancer as primarily artist or technician. When the technical thesis has seemed uppermost rebels have arisen not merely within the ballet, but also outside it; the revolt being either against ballet itself as an art form, as in the case of Duncan, or merely against classical technique as the main component of ballet, as in the case of Jooss. That none of these outside movements has ever seriously affected classical ballet as the principal art form of the dance can be due only to the fact that those equally imbued with the idea of the dancer as an expressive artist have arisen to reform the classical ballet *from within*.

Jooss has merely carried to extremes the principles of Noverre, who wrote of the five positions that "it is the art of the great dancer to neglect them gracefully," of Fokine, who in *Sylphides* showed how the more exaggerated and ugly of the classical effects might be softened to become a means of poetic expression, of Pavlova, perhaps the greatest of all dancer-artists, whose whole career was devoted, in her own words, to making "the physical elements of the dance subservient to the psychological conception." Pavlova was, like Fokine, a romantic in reaction from the virtuosity of pure classicism. Technique for both was not an end in itself, but a means to an end, so successfully achieved in the case of Pavlova that Svetloff wrote of her: "Few are the initiated in choreography who would be able to discern the technical elements in Pavlova's classical dancing. . . . While feeling the brilliant effect

38

of the whole, one cannot grasp the mechanical side or realise the springs of physical elements set in motion to produce this result". Pavlova, by her incomparable range and sensibility, proved to the world that the dancer can be an expressive artist in the genre of Chaliapine in opera and Duse in the theatre. She might well, in fact, have been called "the Duse of the Dance"; the two artists had a great mutual admiration and there is a charming similarity of idiom in Ivor Brown's description of Duse, "our princess of candlelight", and Svetloff's of Pavlova, "the princess of the kingdom of shadows and dreams."

The poetic influence of Fokine and Pavlova on technique has been such that the cold brilliance of the ballerina's traditional style in *Lac des Cygnes*, as exemplified in performances by the Diaghileff and other companies in Europe, has in recent years tended more to the lyrical and tender, especially among English dancers, of whom Margot Fonteyn and Alicia Markova are the outstanding examples. There is no reason why classical ballet rôles, as in the case of classical dramatic rôles such as "Hamlet," should not be open to more than one interpretation, and this softer rendering of Odette is in some ways more justifiable than the other, both as an illustration of the sad romantic spirit of the music and Ivanov's choreography and as a contrast to the harder and more brilliant character, Odile, of Petipa's third Act. In Russia, in fact, where as in England *Lac des Cygnes* is performed in its entirety, the more lyrical interpretation of the second Act is traditional and the great Soviet ballerina, Galina Ulanova, is ranked above her contemporaries mainly because of this poetic quality, which she possesses in addition to the line and technical purity of the Petipa-style ballerina.

But though this increase of lyricism has come to be accepted in the ballerina, her partner is still expected by many merely to reproduce the strength and dazzling technical virtuosity which they imagine, not completely accurately, to be the essence of the *danseur noble*. The Cecchetti tradition in England dies hard, and it is often forgotten that the Italian system of training taught here by this great teacher, and recorded in book form by M. Stanislas Idzikowsky and Mr. Cyril Beaumont, produces great classical technicians but not, by itself, ballerinas and *danseurs noble* of the purest style of the classical ballet. The Russian dancers went to Cecchetti for the added speed, strength and dexterity the Italian school could give their work, but they retained at the same time the grace and more lyrical extended "line" instilled into them by many years' previous training in their own school, developed from the French. "Theirs," writes the Russian teacher Legat of the Italians, "was a school of *tours de force;* taste was sacrificed to effect and dexterity." The tendency in England, where Cecchetti's influence is still very strong, is sometimes to rate the *tours de force* higher than the more important qualities of taste and style, especially among male dancers.

This failure to judge the artist as a whole, and concentration on very minor points of technique, shows a disturbing distortion of relative values. Many balletgoers still seem to have the impression that Pavlova's triumph was based mainly on personality and her technique was faulty, whereas those who watched her most closely at many performances, Svetloff and Levinson among critics and Robert Helpmann among dancers, all agree that her technique was very strong, though she was too great an artist to make it seem at all obvious. The young Helpmann, attached for some time to her company as a student of her partner Novikoff, seems to have been deeply influenced by Pavlova's outlook and it is interesting that of all to-day's dancers his sincerity and range as an artist, as well as his unusual musicality (Andreevsky wrote that Pavlova was "dancing music"), provide perhaps the most obvious parallel to hers. Her advice, "Never take the classroom on to the stage," he has followed to such effect, deliberately avoiding excessive "turning out," which like Pavlova and Fokine he considers inartistic and ugly, and covering every technical feat with a deceptive easy elegance, that many think Helpmann's technical mastery to be much weaker than is actually the case. A sound technical basis, it hardly needs emphasising, is an absolute essential in any dancer, and that Helpmann's technique is equal to the demands of the classical choreography should be obvious from his execution of the double *cabrioles, jetés battus* and *doubles tours en l'air* which make *Giselle* such a test for the *premier danseur.*

That there is still a good deal of misunderstanding about technique and types of dancers is shown by the fact that a recent book by a balletgoer has dismissed Helpmann as not a good classical dancer or, in fact, a *danseur noble* at all, and labelled him as a "character" dancer. This seems to have arisen from the fact that he is a remarkable character *mime,* but for character or national dancing as such he has never shown any special facility—as, for instance, Massine has done. He has not, in fact, the physique or necessary strength of thigh. Like Pavlova, Helpmann is a natural classical dancer who happens also to possess unusual acting ability, though the range in his case is of course wider since it extends to the grotesque.

Most confusion on this point springs from the fact that there are two types of classical male dancers—the *danseur noble* and the *demi-caractère* or virtuoso—and it is a fairly common mistake to expect the first to display the technical speed and facility of the second. Ninette de Valois admirably differentiated the two types in her very clear-headed book, *Invitation to the Ballet*, when she wrote of *demi-caractère* dancers "They possess brilliance, speed and precision as opposed to the lethargy and lyrical musicality which are found in the pure classical performer. The *danseur noble* is the symbol of classical form or creation, the other of classical technique or execution." The essentials of the *danseur noble* are, in fact, nobility of style, great purity of "line" and symmetry of physique, expressiveness as a mime (as hero of the ballet his part is an acting and not purely a dancing one, such as that of the Blue Bird allotted to the virtuoso) and perfect partnering. The following description is also instructive: "He was noted for the extreme artistry of whatever he did. He thought out every rôle in detail. His make-up was marvellous and he possessed a wonderful talent for wearing costume. In addition, he had a remarkable nobility of gesture and elegance of manner and was an excellent and graceful partner. He belonged to the classical dancers of the purest style." This was written not of Helpmann, to whom it applies in every particular, but of Paul Gerdt, teacher of Pavlova and Fokine and a famous *danseur noble* of his time.

Helpmann's academic defects, lack of speed and of strength of beat in the *entrechat*, are the result partly of late training and partly of his physical formation, the perfectly straight legs which give great beauty of "line" but detract from the brilliance of *batterie* achieved by the slight "bow" of the average virtuoso. They are not incompatible with good classical dancing of the *danseur noble* style, and just as Irving's genius overcame his physical defects, including a poor voice, and even turned them into assets, so Helpmann has turned his deficiency, lack of virtuoso strength and pace, into something of far greater value in the artistic sense: exceptional grace, lightness and flow of movement, so that one is never conscious of isolated steps but only of the dance as a whole, not a series of words or even phrases, but a complete poem. No one now denies that Irving was a great actor, and by any serious standards Helpmann must be acknowledged, not the greatest classical technician certainly, but the greatest male *dancer* of his generation, taking the designation of dancer in its highest balletic sense, which includes not only execution but also musical feeling and rhythm, intelligence (a matter of balance and poise in the placing of body and limbs as well as of interpretation), plasticity of facial expression and a wide mimic range. It is the possession of these qualities in an incomparable degree that has placed Helpmann and Massine, his senior by some fifteen years, at the head of all contemporary male dancers. Helpmann has also the very necessary love and feeling for the classical tradition, and the sensitiveness to atmosphere that can help the Princess Aurora to seem an elusive, intangible vision and give to *Sylphides*, at that moment when the male dancer seems to draw the ballerina back across the stage with untouching hands, an unearthly magic. His dancing is the outstanding example of bodily movement controlled and directed by the mind.

Pavlova, like Margot Fonteyn in England to-day, was a born dancer who could never have been anything else; her acting was an indissoluble part of her dance and could hardly have existed without it. Helpmann and Massine are among those rare artists, occurring in every art and headed by Leonardo da Vinci, whose genius is of that many-sided nature that spills itself easily into several mediums. Both are actors and choreographers as much as dancers, and in both cases the early training was dramatic. Massine is the more obvious virtuoso and, unlike Pavlova and Helpmann, in no sense a classical dancer at all; but his virtuosity is based on character and his technique, like theirs, invariably subordinated to the rôle. The truth is, of course, that sheer virtuosity no more makes a great dancer than it makes a great pianist; six *pirouettes à la seconde* turned with unerring style, balance and finish by Helpmann are worth ten by the majority of dancers, and an arabesque or *jeté* by Pavlova worth thirty-two of the *fouettés* her teacher, the wise artist Gerdt, forbade her to attempt. What distinguishes the artist from the virtuoso is an indefinable quality of "style," and its recognition in the classical dancer is particularly essential if standards are not to disintegrate.

The combination of a phenomenal technique with lyricism and true artistry is so rare that Nijinsky appears as something apart, a strange, half-mortal figure, in the history of dancing. Pavlova was probably the greatest of all classical dancers—Levinson wrote of her: "The definition of a modern Taglioni does not appear to me to be sufficient for Pavlova. . . . We have in our midst the greatest dancer of all times, or, to be more exact, of all the historical periods of dancing which admit of analysis"—but it is important to remember that Karsavina equals her in fame as a complete and expressive artist of wide acting range. If Pavlova was the Duse of the dance, Karsavina, perhaps, with her more definitive and passionate characterisation, was the Bernhardt. There is, generally speaking, far too much concentration on footwork, too little on the performance as a whole, among both balletgoers and young dancers, and I should like to see the history of ballet and dancers such as these, "ballet appreciation" in the widest sense, included in the curriculum of all schools of dancing and even secondary schools. Only then, with dancers and balletgoers educated not only in the technical but also in the artistic sense, will the dancer who is also an artist, and the truly discriminating audience, become less rare.

CHAPTER IX

MAKE-UP AND CHARACTER IN BALLET

ONE of the most fascinating aspects of ballet is the study it provides of make-up not only in character but also in purely romantic work. Historical prints of dancers, in which the emphasis is mainly on costume or those fantastically attenuated *pointes* beloved of the lithographer, suggest that early ballet make-up was largely naturalistic and differed little from that of actors and actresses in the dramatic theatre. It was possibly the orientation of ballet from France and Italy to Russia that led finally to the more stylised and exotic make-up used by the dancers of most companies, English and Russian, to-day.

There is, of course, a danger in this exoticism, and pictures from America suggest that there glamorisation has tended to overbalance in the direction of Hollywood. Too heavy a make-up is fatal to the spirit of a ballet such as *Sylphides*, and even in modern and classical work false eyelashes, "hot-black" applied to the lashes, rouge and those small slanting lines at the outside corners of the eyes that give such a fascinating touch of stylisation to ballet make-up are only completely effective if applied with artistry and restraint. This is especially important in parts such as Giselle and the Young Girl in *Spectre de la Rose*, where any hint of sophistication destroys the character. Margot Fonteyn's make-up, with the large dark eyes that are, as an actress, her most valuable physical asset emphasised by a slight touch of red and a delicately pale make-up of the face, is ideal for these parts, though of course different facial constructions and colourings require different treatment. Fonteyn uses "hot-black" but not false eyelashes; some eyes need this extra emphasis, but it inclines to veil the eyes too heavily if these are small and narrow in shape.

Generally speaking the ballerina is not called upon for much variety of character make-up, and even the average *demi-caractère danseuse* rarely has to cope with any more complicated make-up than that of the Doll in *Petrouchka;* though a painstaking artist will sometimes take the trouble to build up, say, a more suitable nose, as Baronova

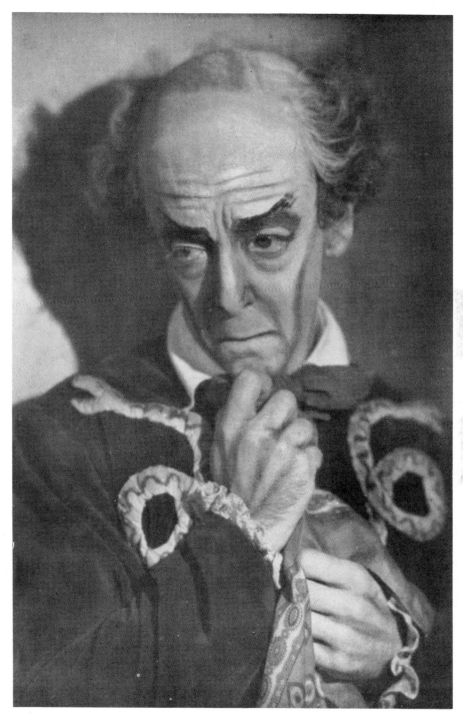

Make-up and Character
Robert Helpmann as Dr. Coppelius

Plate XI

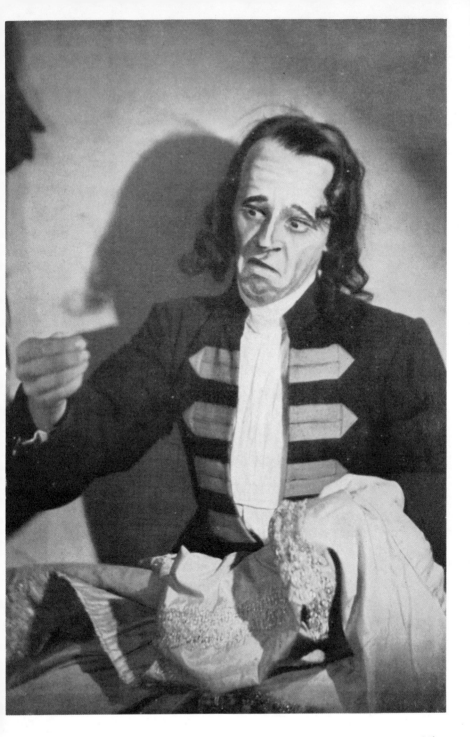

Make-up and Character
Ray Powell as the Tailor in *The Rake's Progress*

Plate XII

did for the part of Lady Gay in *Union Pacific*, and certain parts, such as the Fox in Andrée Howard's ballet, require a very specialised make-up, which Sally Gilmour achieves in the auburn-coloured slant of the eyes, repeating the effect of the hair, dressed into two little points like animal's ears.

In a ballet such as *The Rake's Progress* every part is a "character" part and each of its eighteenth-century drabs, with blotted-out teeth and raddled dishevelment, requires an individual make-up. Ray Powell's Tailor was a remarkable example of face-building in this ballet, in which the sagging grooves of the skin, embedded with the grit of eighteenth-century London, and the contemptuous droop of the mouth pointed a definite and sourly fawning character. This very young dancer's gift for make-up and characterisation was also shown in his old German tutor in *Lac des Cygnes* and his more roving-eyed ancient in *Promenade*. Each of his old men was different and his training as an artist probably helped him to conceive and execute these dissimilar faces. There is no doubt a talent for drawing, or at least a knowledge and appreciation of art, helps the character dancer no less than the choreographer. Helpmann has said that before attempting his characterisation of the Rake he studied the faces in Hogarth's original pictures with a magnifying glass, which may explain why his skin in the Lunatic scene has the effect of the pigmentation, that faint iridescent blend of amethyst and green, in a portrait in oils. His whole make-up scheme in *The Rake's Progress* combines with his acting to reveal the gradual degeneration of the character. Already in the Orgy scene the lines of the face are beginning to sag in dissipation, and there are ugly bags under the eyes. In the Card scene only the dregs of elegance remain, the face is unshaven, vicious, the twitching mouth and nerveless hands anticipating the madness of the following scene, where the eyes have become raw-rimmed and lashless and the face, shrunk and wasted by disease, seems the more poignant for the sinister, bleeding gash in the cheek.

The colour and design of the costume are, of course, frequent guides to the type of make-up required, and how the artist's intention may be defeated by inadequate make-up is shown by a comparison of the face in John Piper's original design for "Lechery" in *The Quest* with that seen on the stage in performance. The ape-like repulsion of Piper's design could, perhaps, only successfully be produced in a mask, and Gordon Hamilton's deliberately static and unreal make-up for "Avarice," with heavy bronze-green lips and eyelids, was effective mainly for its mask-like quality. The colour of the costume may be very effectively echoed in a touch of make-up; Alexis Rassine's blue eyelids as the Dove in *The Birds* were a case in point.

In comic parts ballet make-up usually tends to caricature. Massine's clown-white face, tousled black hair and moustache in *Boutique Fantasque* and *Union Pacific* had a Chaplinesque impertinence; Helpmann as Mr. O'Reilly and Dr. Coppelius also favours the clown touch, though in his case the creation is more individual, its partial derivative being the Harlequinade make-up of the Grimaldi tradition. The green half-moons under the eyes combine with the red nose and thin slit of mouth, curving upwards or downwards at will, to give to Mr. O'Reilly a watery drunken cheerfulness or glumness, and in Dr. Coppelius one senses throughout, in the gait and pucker of the mouth, a real old man beneath the caricature. The basic make-up before the caricature is added is, indeed, that of a realistic ancient, shrivelled and yellow of skin, and the transformation from nonagenarian to clown is fascinating to watch.

Helpmann's face is naturally plastic and transformable and falls easily into the lines of Dr. Coppelius, which make-up, though it looks so much more elaborate, is in fact much quicker to complete than that of Hamlet, where the eyelashes have to be painstakingly applied with "hot-black," the skin given a cream-like smoothness and the curve of lips and eyebrows drawn with extreme care. Out of the theatre lights this make-up, with its buff-coloured basis, violet eyelids and vermilion mouth, has a fantastic beauty. It is instructive to compare it with Helpmann's make-up in *Hamlet* the play, a purely realistic conception in which eyes, lips and skin were only very lightly touched up. Yet curiously ballet creates its own convention of realism, and the contrast of this with that of the dramatic theatre was interestingly shown when for one performance of *The Quest*, in response to a suggestion, Helpmann appeared in the part of St. George practically without make-up, as if for a play. The result was ineffective and even, in the balletic surroundings, unnatural.

Actually Helpmann's career provides an interesting example of gradual enhancement of facial possibilities. In his early ballet appearances his small and curiously mediæval face, with its expressive but unnaturally large round eyes and parted lips, gave all his stage characters an individual and Puckish quality, charming but immature. Later he learned to lengthen the eyes, to give a firmer and graver contour to the mouth, with the result that in romantic parts the whole face has taken on character and dignity. This is of course due in some part to increased maturity, and like everything else where an actor's work is concerned make-up is only half the battle, the mental approach of the artist to the rôle being equally important. Massine, for instance, permits himself the flippancy of curled eyebrows in *Gaieté Parisienne*, but otherwise the characterisation of the Peruvian depends entirely on the playing; similarly in *The Three-Cornered Hat* his essentially Spanish portrayal is a matter not of make-up but of temperament vividly suggested in the flash of eye and teeth and the movement of the whole body. In the case of outstanding artists acting can transform their entire appearance. It was written of Edmund Kean, according to Macready "a little, mean-looking man," that as Othello "he seemed to *expand* from a small, resolute figure and assume the vigour and dimensions of a giant." Helpmann similarly as Satan in *Job* seems to grow in physique by sheer force of acting, for the additional dominating power of his naturally slender frame is certainly only in part due to the elaborate all-over make-up of the body, in which the muscles, as in a Blake engraving, are outlined in greasepaint. The baleful and dæmonic effect of his eye make-up for this part, slanted in red and green streaks towards the temples, is also accentuated by the concentrated evil of the expression.

How useless make-up may be without emotional feeling and sense of character behind it has been shown in several cases in ballet where a second player has taken up a part with the identical make-up of his or her predecessor, and yet has seemed entirely ineffectual in comparison. Martin Harvey wrote of Irving: "I have seen, in the death throes of the old tyrant, Louis XI, his eyes positively glaze as the *rigor mortis* froze into immobility the hands which he stretched forth to clutch his crown for the last time." Make-up in a case such as this becomes irrelevant; only acting of genius could achieve the effect. "The only real secret," in Helpmann's own words, "is *sincerity*."

THE ENGLISH SCENE

CHAPTER X

SADLER'S WELLS : THE ENGLISH NATIONAL BALLET

IN Chapter III reference has been made to the startling rise in popularity of ballet since the war, and the formation of new companies ostensibly presenting "ballet" but in most cases losing title to serious consideration because of their choreographic or dancing poverty and lack of traditional background. Such companies served their turn in war-time as providers of entertainment and spectacle for theatregoers with no previous knowledge of ballet; but lacking artistic roots and background they will, unless their policy and standards are seriously overhauled, inevitably disappear when the present "boom" ends. Ballet then will survive through those companies who have, over a period of years, built on a sound basis of knowledge and integrity and have shown consistent development. This means, in England, and omitting such alien growths as the Ballets Jooss and whatever foreign companies may visit us after the war, the Sadler's Wells Company and the Ballet Rambert.

In January 1945 the Sadler's Wells Company, sponsored by E.N.S.A., went on a prolonged tour of the Continent, playing both in garrison and public theatres in Brussels and Paris with a repertoire of nine ballets, most of them English works which were originally produced for this company by its own choreographers and which have placed English ballet on an artistic level with the famous Russian companies which visited us before the war. These ballets represented but a proportion of the total English repertoire created by this company and the Ballet Rambert since their formation, and it is difficult to believe that less than twenty years ago there was no such thing as English ballet outside the music hall, to which all our dancers who did not take up teaching or enter foreign companies were forced to gravitate.

English ballet received its first impetus several years before the death of Diaghileff in 1929, when Marie Rambert began to train

English dancers in a school from which many notable future choreo-graphers and designers were also to emerge, and from which her own intimate ballet company shortly afterwards evolved. Almost simul-taneously—in 1926—Ninette de Valois, a young dancer with choreographic ambitions and a gift for organisation, had opened an Academy of Choreographic Art in London, a short-lived enterprise which was to prove the prelude to a greater achievement. For the Sadler's Wells Ballet, now the major English company, had its beginnings as a self-sufficient entity in 1931, when the late Lilian Baylis reopened the Sadler's Wells Theatre as a home for opera and ballet and a sister theatre to the Old Vic, in which she had already established a successful policy of presenting Shakespeare "for the people." There was already a nucleus ballet company in the six dancers of the Old Vic Opera Company, for which Miss Baylis had engaged Ninette de Valois to produce the ballets some while previously, and the opening of Sadler's Wells gave this small nucleus the necessary opportunities for expansion and development.

Within a few years the Sadler's Wells Ballet was a full-scale company of international reputation, with a repertoire of classical ballets and major home-produced works and a thriving school of ballet in which some of its best dancers—including its young ballerina, Margot Fonteyn—had been trained. In 1937 they were invited to represent English ballet at the Paris Exhibition, and in 1940 they were on a British Council tour of Holland when the Nazi invasion forced them to flee from a frontier town at a few hours' notice, leaving all the effects of their ballets behind them, a loss that by 1945 they had still not entirely made good. Since the "blitz" of 1940 drove the company from their original home they have built up large new audiences in the provinces and in the West End, where, in spite of the shortage of male dancers, which weakened performances of some ballets and made a few impossible to produce (upwards of a score of Wells dancers have served in the Forces), they have added to their repertoire a number of fine and lasting works and given two four-act Russian classical ballets, the Petipa–Tchaikovsky *Lac des Cygnes* and *The Sleeping Beauty*, brilliant new productions.

The question as to whether the Sadler's Wells Ballet or the Ballet Rambert, after a decade or more of existence, can be more truly termed the English National Ballet could hardly have arisen in an art less permeated by partisanship and "behind scenes" politics than that of ballet. No music lover or musician would seriously apply the title of

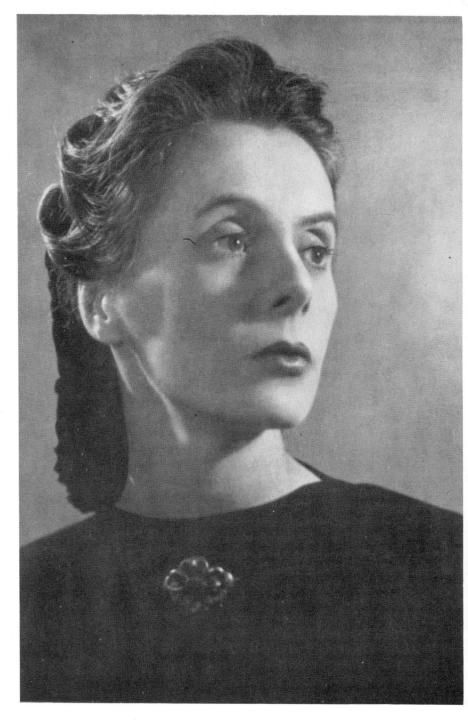

Ninette de Valois

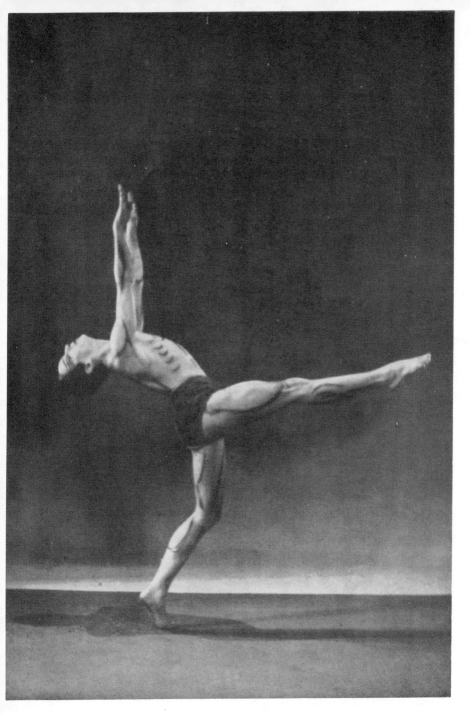

Photo   *Anthony*

Job
Satan's Dance: Robert Helpmann

Plate XIV

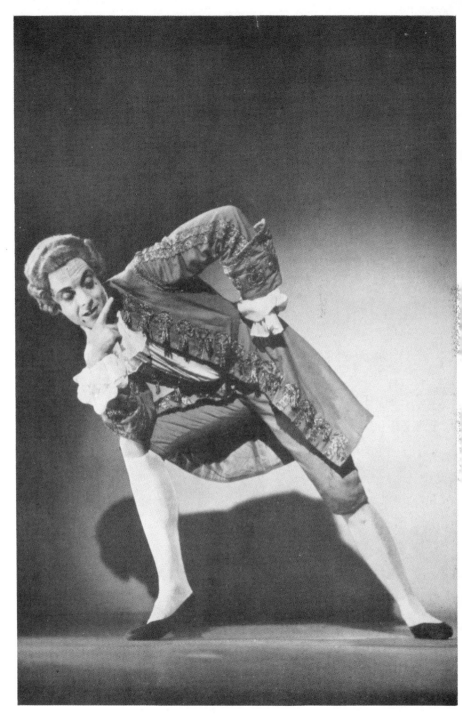

The Rake's Progress
Robert Helpmann as the Rake

Plate XV

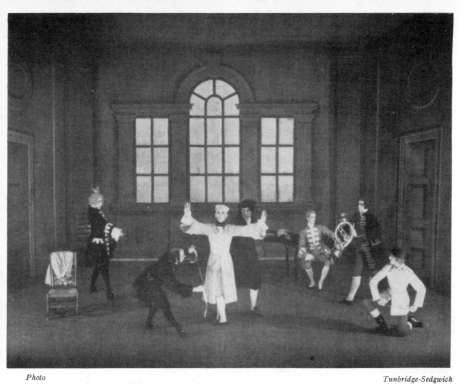

Photo

Tunbridge-Sedgwick

Plate XVI   (*Above*) *The Rake's Progress:* Opening Scene
Designs after Hogarth by Rex Whistler

Plate XVII   (*Below*) Death of the Rake (Robert Helpmann)

Action Photo

G. B. L. Wilson

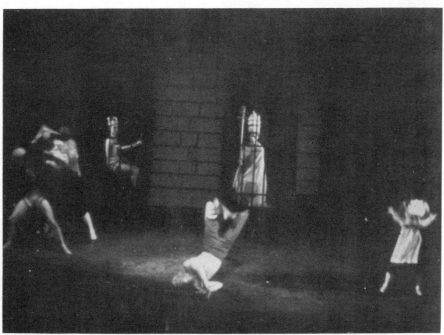

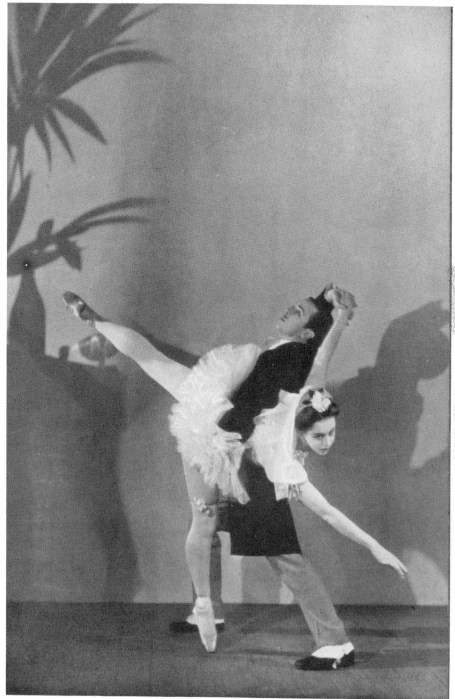

Comedy (Ashton): *The Wedding Bouquet*
Pas de Deux: Mary Honer and Robert Helpmann

Plate XVIII

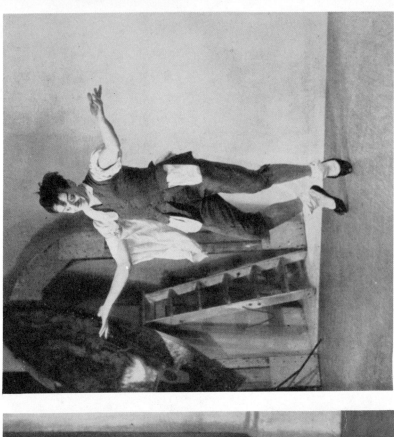

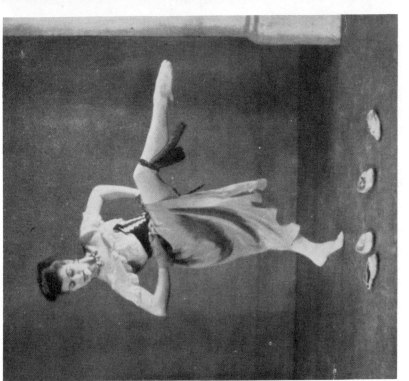

Comedy (de Valois): *The Prospect Before Us*

Ballerina's Dance: Julia Farron

Mr. O'Reilly's Dance: Robert Helpmann

Plate XIX

Plate XX

"National Orchestra" to a chamber music quintet, however high its standards of playing and repertoire; in every country in which the fine arts—music, ballet or the drama—are subsidised by the State the term "National" automatically implies an organised body capable of performing major full-scale works both modern and classical. The Ballet Rambert has never yet been able, by reason of its restricted size, to maintain classical works on an adequate scale in its repertoire, and its best choreographers have created their most important ballets after leaving the company to work within larger organisations such as Sadler's Wells and the Ballet Theatre of America.

The term "National" has also other and more material implications. It implies permanency, freedom from the profit-making motive, if possible an attached school, directorship elastically controlled by an impartial governing body. How fatal dependency on one individual and private enterprise can be to the survival of a ballet company has been shown by the complete disintegration of the Diaghileff Ballet after his death and, more recently, by a tragic enforced break of two years in the existence of the Ballet Rambert. The Sadler's Wells Company, attached to the Old Vic organisation which in England most nearly approximates in conditions to a National Theatre, is free from this precariousness of existence; it has its own ballet school and permanent company, it is independent of ordinary commercial "backing," and because of its sound planning and background it would survive, even though it would temporarily suffer by, a change of directorship.

The Sadler's Wells Ballet holds its pre-eminent position in England not only because it has kept the major classical ballets in its repertoire (apart from Diaghileff's short-lived production of *The Sleeping Princess* in London in 1921 it is, in fact, the only ballet company outside Russia regularly to perform this ballet and *Lac des Cygnes* in their entirety), but because the best native choreographers and (with few exceptions) dancers work for it. No English choreographers, Helpmann perhaps apart, seriously compare in stature and achievement with Frederick Ashton and Ninette de Valois, and their greatest ballets —*Apparitions, Horoscope, Dante Sonata, The Wanderer, Job, The Rake's Progress, Checkmate*—have all been created for the Wells or (in the case of *Job*, created for the Camargo Society which in England productively bridged the gap between the death of Diaghileff and the establishment of a permanent English company) absorbed into its repertoire. Margot Fonteyn and Robert Helpmann are equally indisputably the leading dancers in England and artistically they rank with those of any foreign company seen here. Apart from Marie Rambert (a fine inspirer of talent but not herself a creator), the main influence on English ballet has been exercised by Ninette de Valois, Frederick Ashton and Robert Helpmann. Ninette de Valois takes first place not only because the Sadler's Wells Ballet is in every important sense her own creation, but because more than any English choreographer she has given to native ballet an atmosphere and character of its own. Ashton has added the brilliance of dance invention which was necessary if English ballet was to preserve its link with classical tradition, together with increasing emotional depth and poetic imagery. Helpmann's influence as a choreographer has hardly had time to crystallise (although the original dramatic impact of his major works is certain to be felt in the future); but as a dancer-mime of outstanding genius he has had an obvious and valuable influence in shaping the dramatic trend of English choreography and in inspiring other dancers by his artistry and sincerity. Constant Lambert's work as musical director of the Wells has also been of unique value to English ballet, and with ballet scores by such contemporary composers as Lambert himself, Arthur Bliss, William Walton and Vaughan Williams, as well as discriminating taste in the selection and arrangement of existing music, the musical record of this company is unequalled since the time of Diaghileff. As regards *décor* the Wells has employed many fine artists and Leslie Hurry, a Helpmann discovery, is the major figure in ballet design of recent years.

It would be uncritical not to admit that these major achievements have been matched by some minor failures of policy and creation, inevitable under the war-time strain of giving eight performances a week in addition to the classes and constant rehearsal necessary to maintain a score of old and new ballets in the repertoire. There is a tendency to put promising young *danseuses* into exacting parts before they are technically or mentally fully equipped for them, and to perform some ballets, particularly the classics, too frequently with an inferior cast. The policy of "two or three dancers, one part," advocated by Arnold Haskell in his admirable recent book on the Wells, *National Ballet*, is justifiable only if "two or three dancers" of a style and technique truly adequate for the part are available. There was a relatively brief period, too, in the latter part of the war when three consecutive new productions, in which neither of the company's two principal dancers appeared, were of so light a texture thematically that the need for a new ballet of more dramatic stamina began very definitely to be felt.

The last of these three works, *Le Festin de l'Araignée* by Andrée Howard, has some historical importance as the first ballet since the company's earliest days to be created for the Wells by an "outside" choreographer (Miss Howard had been attached for some months to the Sadler's Wells Ballet School but her main work has been for the Ballet Rambert). The music, a fascinating score originally composed for a ballet of the same name at the Paris Opera, was by Roussel, and the *décor* and costumes by Michael Ayrton, a young artist whose designs, dominated by a gigantic spider's web, had sinister imagination and a richness of colouring not previously attained in his easel and theatre work. Unfortunately the ballet was not up to the standard of its production and this was in the main due to the lack of any dramatic or character interest in the theme. The spectacle of insects devouring one another can yield nothing but horror unless, as in *The Insect Play*, there is a bitter and satiric human parallelism. Without the character development of Miss Howard's earlier *Lady Into Fox* or the humour and parody of Helpmann's *The Birds* the insect or animal ballet can only be optical and there is nothing on which the mind or sympathies can fasten. The failure of this ballet, which was below the choreographic standard of Miss Howard's previous work, marked, however, the end of this overlight period of creation. Helpmann's *Miracle in the Gorbals* and a revival of Ashton's *Nocturne* soon afterwards magnificently restored the balance, and the list of new productions by the Sadler's Wells Ballet over the whole period of the war exceeds in creative quality that of any English company and probably any Russian-American. It shows, in fact, a progressive choreographic achievement that would be remarkable even in peace-time.

That English ballet, in the few years of its existence, has been able to produce dancers of the status of Fonteyn and Helpmann, choreographers of the individuality and power of de Valois, Ashton and Helpmann, and a musical director, Constant Lambert, who has no equal in ballet anywhere to-day—in addition to a supporting company in which a talent for character and drama, as well as for dancing, is rapidly maturing—is a confirmation of Diaghileff's prophecy that the English would one day play a predominant part in the world of ballet. In the middle of the most terrible and devastating war in history Sadler's Wells was still able to show to foreign countries a truly creative national ballet of which England could be proud, and the shift to Covent Garden in 1946, together with the formation of the second company at Sadler's Wells, marked a new and important phase in English ballet history.

CHAPTER XI

THE BALLETS OF NINETTE DE VALOIS

A LARGE part of the credit for this progression of the Sadler's Wells Ballet under war-time hazards is due to the foresight and driving genius of Ninette de Valois. An Irish dancer who had been a soloist in Diaghileff's Russian company and learned every aspect of stage production, dramatic as well as balletic, at such theatres as the Abbey, Dublin, and the Arts, Cambridge, her achievement as founder and director of what is, in effect, the English National Ballet has seemed to overshadow in some minds her importance as a choreographer. With *Job* and *The Rake's Progress* now both, after a war-time absence, in the Sadler's Wells repertoire, it must be apparent even to newcomers to ballet that Miss de Valois's work as choreographer has been of equal significance. She has not merely founded a ballet school and practising company; she has given to English choreography, as has been seen, a new and vital direction and characteristic. In the history of ballet she must stand as the first great English choreographer, and in the national sense she retains her pre-eminence to-day beside the more Russian-grounded genius of Ashton, the dramatically vibrant but as yet unprolific Helpmann, and the sometimes overrated but exceptionally talented Antony Tudor, some of whose small ballets produce a curiously Gallic effect of style, but a major work by whom has yet to be seen in England.

JOB

JOB, the first great ballet to reveal a definite national style, has therefore historical as well as artistic importance. It is great not only in choreography but also in music and inspiration. Blake's illustrations to the Book of Job, a unique mystical manifestation in English art, have provided the choreographer with a foundation on which, with the help of Gwendoline Raverat's settings and thunder-red drop curtain, she has built a ballet remarkable not only for its quality of pliant grouping but of mind. *Job* is a spiritual experience; an effect heightened by the grave, ritualistic pattern of the Hebrew dances and the dramatic stylisation of the masked figure of God (confusingly designated in the programme as "Job's Spiritual Self," an ambiguity which could only be necessary in an age as religiously weak-kneed as our own). It is also superb drama, the choreographer and scenarist, Geoffrey Keynes, having vividly realised the action implicit behind the theological argument and imagery of the Bible story, and created the ballet around the epic theme of Satan's ambition pitched against the power of God. The power of thought and ideology cannot be translated adequately into movement; but Victor Hugo had a similar sense of this integral motive power behind the Book of Job when he wrote in his *William Shakespeare*[1]: "Job begins the drama . . . by placing Jehovah and Satan in presence of each other; the evil defies the good and behold! action is begun." It is by the selection of this theatric element in *Job* as the basis of the ballet, and Ninette de Valois's translation of Blake's vision into simple, plastic groupings which have the effect of animated pictures, that the choice of theme has been justified. Vaughan Williams's music, the best yet composed for an English ballet, matches Blake in robustness and serenity, and in the dance of Satan takes on a barbaric quality, stabbing and hesitant in rhythm, which Miss de Valois has paralleled in movement with virile imagination. This solo, an exciting study of primitive evil, is now danced by Robert Helpmann with a fine appreciation of its savagery and subtle rhythm.

Satan is Miss de Valois's supreme creation, and the dramatic climaxes of the ballet centre in him; in his rebellious demand of God, the withering malediction of his outflung arm marking Job as his prey, his triumphant mounting of the throne of God, his headlong fall in defeat. It is a rôle that demands quite exceptional dramatic and musical powers in the performer. Created by Anton Dolin as a figure of splendid physical pride, it is only since Robert Helpmann took over the character that it has acquired its full preternatural virulence of body and mind. This is a Prince of Darkness of Miltonic arrogance, who might cry as in *Paradise Lost*, "Better to reign in hell than serve in heaven"! The very contraction of the back muscles as this Satan kneels before the throne suggests bitter humiliation and

[1] A study of Æschylus, Homer, Job, Juvenal, Lucretius, Dante, Michaelangelo, Rembrandt, Rabelais, Beethoven and others, and a triumph of discursiveness at which the most famous of our present-day dramatic critics might well pale.

defiance, and seated on the throne itself, like a statue by Michaelangelo in green bronze, he has a livid and destructive malevolence. Hazlitt wrote of Kean's Richard III that it "filled every part of the stage," and Helpmann's Satan does, indeed, seem to grow both physically and mentally, and fill the stage with a sense of frustrated power. The almost lay figure of Job requires an actor who can make stillness positive, if it is to have any significance, and this rare gift unfortunately does not belong to small-part actors; but in the revival of this ballet at the New Theatre in December 1943 the team-work was notable, David Paltenghi's Elihu caught the Apollo-like brightness and poignancy of "Ye are old, and I am very young," and Celia Franca's ebony and ivory beauty, in a dress like a green flame, made a centrepiece to the pictures of Hebraic loveliness.

LA CRÉATION DU MONDE : THE HAUNTED BALLROOM

J O B was the one great work in the earliest Sadler's Wells programmes, a herald of what English ballet might achieve in the future, although the necessity to create a repertoire from scratch meant at the time a preponderance of hastily-conceived works with, in the main, little stamina for survival. Two of Ninette de Valois's ballets in this period were, however, of more substantial quality. The theme and music (by Darius Milhaud) of *La Création du Monde* were taken from a production by the short-lived but creative Swedish Ballet at the Theatre des Champs-Élysées, Paris, in 1923, the original choreography being by Jean Borlin. Ninette de Valois gave to her version the quality of a negro ritual, in which life was generated from the massed confusion before Creation by the incantations of three primitive gods. Silhouetted starkly against the background, these figures both in their staccato choreographic movement and the fantastic costumes and masks designed by Edward Wolfe had something of the effect of the three figures of War, Pestilence and Famine in *Job*. The emergence of plant and animal life from primæval chaos, and its culmination in the creation of Man and Woman, formed a choreographic study of extraordinary vividness and originality at that time, and although the ballet has not been revived for many years it would almost certainly take its place in the repertoire to-day without seeming below the general choreographic level of the company. The negro spiritual atmosphere of the revival scene in Robert Helpmann's *Miracle in the Gorbals* is, in fact, the only English ballet scene produced since of anything like the same genre, though the substitution of a modern slum for the primitive setting gives a totally different angle to the effect.

The Haunted Ballroom, the next most important work by Ninette de Valois of this period, is historically interesting in that the character of the Master of Treginnis provided the young Robert Helpmann with his first created part. Though not, as has erroneously been stated, based on a story by Edgar Allan Poe, the mental atmosphere created by that superb essayist in the macabre was reproduced in this ballet through mime, dance and music. The first scene, entirely in mime, prepared the stage for the strange tragedy of the second, in which the Master of the house, drawn sleeping into the fatal ballroom where his ancestors had mysteriously perished, was danced to death by ghostly revellers led by the Paganini-like figure of a sinister flautist. The division of the ballet into one scene of mime and one of dance unbalanced it as an entity; but the music of Geoffrey Toye, the "Motley" designs and the choreography, with its menacing lines and groups and its misty suggestion of untouchability in the spirits, created together an impression which had something of the fateful inevitability of *The Fall of the House of Usher*. The ballet was beautifully rounded off by the poignant comment of its final picture: the small son of the dead Master alone on the stage with a sudden fearful realisation of his own destiny. This part in 1934 was mimed with an arresting sensitivity by a dark-eyed, fifteen-year-old child from the *corps de ballet* who, in the intermediate agonies of rechristening, called herself Margot Fontes. The part of Alicia, the woman guest of the first scene who in the second takes the form of the ghostly seductive leader of the dance of death, was created for Alicia Markova, whose elegance and ethereal lightness fitted it to perfection. In the revivals Margot Fonteyn has acted and danced it with a sensitive feeling for atmosphere and beautiful style and control, and it has also been charmingly mimed by Julia Farron, although this dancer lacks the natural spirituality and *ballon* for the second scene. Pamela May, less sympathetic in the mime, has danced the ghostly episodes with a frigid remoteness that was strangely effective, substituting enticement and terror for actual intangibility. Helpmann's strongly imagined sense of fatality in the leading rôle pervaded the whole ballet and first made obvious his future as a dramatic mime of striking and individual quality. His dancing of the solo in this ballet has always been a remarkable example of grace and musical continuity of line.

THE RAKE'S PROGRESS

IT was with *The Rake's Progress*, however, that Ninette de Valois consolidated her achievement in *Job*, and the production of this ballet in 1935 (with Walter Gore and Markova in the parts to which Helpmann and Elizabeth Miller very shortly afterwards succeeded) marked the beginning of a rich creative period in English ballet.

The Rake's Progress, based on the series of morality pictures by Hogarth, is a great ballet not only in the sense that it is artistically complete and vividly self-explanatory, but also because it remains the best example to date of a balletic style that is essentially English, a style that brings ballet back to the theatre where it traditionally belongs, and realises the special strength of the English dancer, the ability to mime and create character. The Hogarthian atmosphere of this ballet could have been reproduced in no other country; it has an eighteenth-century gusto in which wit, satire, raffishness and stark horror are dramatically balanced and in which every character is sharply etched. Hazlitt, in an essay on the paintings of Hogarth, pointed out that his faces go to the very verge of caricature and yet never go beyond it; and Ninette de Valois has achieved the same sense of life so heightened in intensity that it only just keeps on what Shakespeare's Beatrice would call "the windy side" of caricature. There are inspired details, among them the first picture of the Rake ringed with parasites and being measured, in dance, by the Tailor; the reluctance of the Betrayed Girl, half-petulant, half-sad, and the bristling vengefulness of the Mother; the dance of the two drabs, prinking their hair with a ghastly coquettry; the genuinely funny musicians and the way in which the Singer, succumbing to the temptations of the Orgy, briskly gets rid of her two disapproving accompanists (John Field's trombonist in the 1942 revival was, one suspected, a prop of the local Evangelist band); the creditors impatiently taking snuff astride their chairs; the witty balletic conception of the card game with its mounting undercurrent of terror; the pitiful dance of the girl and the whole macabre pattern of the Lunatic scene, comparable to the less tragic Asylum scene in *Peer Gynt* which Robert Helpmann has arranged for the Old Vic Drama Company with something the same impression of fantastic realism. The introduction of the fashionable women visitors in this scene, frivolous and unmoved, is a biting social comment, and the distorted glance back to the Card scene in the forlorn turned-in figure of the Rake's friend, and the playing of a madman with a rope that seems to have become to him a thing snake-like, sinister and alive, are drawn with a curious insight, humane yet brutally exact. The choreographer is helped by Gavin Gordon's music, an ideal ballet score which is at once danceable and dramatic, and by Rex Whistler's Hogarthian costumes and beautifully-drawn drop curtain.

The Rake's Progress was one of the ballets lost in Holland in 1940. It was revived at the New Theatre on 27th October 1942, when the young company rose to the production with a quite surprising assurance in characterisation and dance, Gordon Hamilton giving an unexpectedly neat execution of Harold Turner's original part of the Dancing Master, and combining it with a performance of the Man with the Rope which gained steadily in force and macabre detail. Ray Powell's Tailor, Joy Newton's Singer and the drabs of Moyra Fraser and Celia Franca were also completely in the Hogarth picture, and Mary Honer gave a lovely performance as the Girl, realising exactly where satire ends and true feeling begins, and infusing into the last scene a wounded and wistful loyalty that was deeply touching. In the dance with the embroidery, Ninette de Valois's most lyrical piece of choreography, her hands had true eloquence. "A face needs hands to give expression to the whole portrait" wrote Leonardo da Vinci, and watching this performance, and Robert Helpmann's in the Card scene, one understood what he meant. Mary Honer's performance remains the criterion for this part. It is the only character of which Margot Fonteyn, an exquisite interpreter of Ashton's ballets and the classical rôles, has not yet completely got the measure, although since her first performance, when she unbalanced the satiric first scene by making us too conscious of the Girl's tragedy, she has attained a stronger sense of the Hogarthian atmosphere and the necessary opening touch of woebegone silliness. The part has rarely been danced with such lightness and precision, although her sewing in the embroidery dance, with tightly-clenched fingers, tends to destroy the delicate grace of the hand movements. The part has also been charmingly played by Mavis Jackson and Julia Farron, the last a beautifully-sustained characterisation proceeding from prettiness to tragic awareness, and the best thing this excellent young *demi-caractère* dancer has yet given us.

Helpmann's Rake dominates the ballet. It remains a penetrating study in degeneracy, gathering in momentum from the first enjoyment of new-found wealth and sowing of wild oats to the Nemesis-haunted

Card scene and desolation of the madhouse, in which even the outward glamour of rakedom is stripped bare to reveal a creature broken, half-animal, pitiable alike in its trapped hopelessness and mad, twitching face. For it is the special strength of Helpmann's acting that, without mitigating the horror, it forces one to accept the Girl's protective love for this battered and hardly human wreck. The Rake is a part that demands tragic acting as the dramatic theatre understands that term and Helpmann alone of modern dancers is able to provide this. The ballet, a masterpiece, exists without him; but it is a less shattering and infinitely less moving experience.

THE PROSPECT BEFORE US

NINETTE DE VALOIS has shown throughout her career the sensitive response to painting, and genius for translating its essence into the moving picture of choreography, that Helpmann has shown to English drama. In *Job* and *The Rake's Progress* she has galvanised Blake and Hogarth to motion with astonishing force and imagination, and in *The Prospect Before Us* she has captured the frothy ebullience of Rowlandson's caricatures with equal facility. That the ballet cannot rank with *The Rake's Progress* is due to the fact that the scenes and story are less cogent and well-knit than in that extremely compact masterpiece. In *Rake* there is not a movement which seems redundant or is not vividly expressive. In *Prospect* one whole scene—that with the lawyers—could be removed without loss to the progression of the story and little to the choreography; all it has to say is or could be telescoped into Mr. O'Reilly's following dance in front of the drop curtain. The lawyers themselves lack the character and inventiveness of their opposites in *Rake*, the creditors, and the dances of Mr. O'Reilly and his rival theatre manager, Mr. Taylor, in front of the curtain are also considerably less interesting than those of the Dancing Master and the Girl in the earlier ballet.

It is, however, necessary for the critic to keep his head and realise that minor defects do not prevent this being a first-class piece of foolery and re-creation of period. The first scene ballet rehearsal is a brilliant and mature choreographic expression of a subject Ashton has also treated, more immaturely, in his early Dégas ballet, *Foyer de Danse*. In its witty observation of character and dance, its little cross-currents of quarrel, reconciliation, boredom and artistic temperament, this scene is an amused and amusing commentary beautiful in its completeness. The eighteenth-century flavour is also cleverly evoked in the urchin-infested street scene and the "ballet within a ballet," which manages to preserve a period charm even while deliciously parodying the dramatic inanities against which Noverre rose in revolt. And in Mr. O'Reilly, the theatre manager of fluctuating fortunes and sobriety, Miss de Valois has created one of the great comic figures in ballet in our time, with a final variation which ranks with Massine's absurdly eccentric Cake Walk in *Union Pacific*.

The Irish have an amiable gift for debunking themselves as well as everyone else, and Miss de Valois's irrepressible tippler is a "darlin' man" of O'Casey-like vintage, though (perhaps significant of Irish womanhood, continually on the pull against male irresponsibility) without the gloss of lyrical moonshine with which Irish male dramatists invest their Paycocks and Playboys. Robert Helpmann's brimming invention in this part showed signs in the 1943 revival of having been dammed (I hope I am correct in spelling the word with an "m") by authority; this is good for the ballet, or not, according to whether one considers the part in this case greater than the whole. Certainly the choreographer owes as much to the interpreter as the interpreter to the choreographer, and the performance of this born clown remains a touchstone of drollery. Max Beerbohm, writing inimitably of Henry Irving, said "comedy comes out of the actor's own soul." If this is true the great comedian will reflect something of the sadness as well as the gaiety within him, for artists are not, generally speaking, completely happy men. Perhaps this is why the greatest clowns, Leno and Chaplin, have pathos as well as humour, and the little crabbed apple of a face Helpmann has built himself for this part is wistful as well as comic. In any event this is an expert piece of comedy timing, every mood caught in a glum droop of the mouth, a disconsolate shrug, a beam of blissful intoxication; and in the final burlesque of a ballerina ridiculousness touches a reeling apex.

Pamela May was the creator of the part of the ballerina when the ballet was first produced in 1940, and since her return to the company following a long absence she has once again given it her quick wit and mimicry. Julia Farron, always an intelligent and vivacious actress, danced and mimed the part in the revival with charming insouciance, and looked so pretty that Rowlandson, watching from his artist's heaven, must have felt envious that she, instead of the original Mlle Theodore, was not the model for his picture. Margaret Dale's Cupid, precise and saucy, was equally attractive. The dancer playing Vestris

is faced with the frightening task of emulating the dancing powers of
the Nijinsky of his age; Alexis Rassine went to it with supple agility
and much improved neatness of finish, and depicted the off-hand
tantrums of a leading man with unexpected wit and style. The still
more formidable task of putting Noverre on to the stage might be
said to have defeated the choreographer before she started. Frederick
Ashton's saturnine aristocrat in the original production more nearly
suggested the "Shakespeare of the Dance" than Ray Powell's later
study, though this was an intelligent piece of mime by a young dancer,
then under twenty, who before his call-up showed signs of becoming
one of the best character mimes this company has yet produced.
Gordon Hamilton also proved himself a worthy successor to Claude
Newman as Mr. Taylor, a modest small portrait that managed to be a
little more than Mr. O'Reilly's "stooge."

Constant Lambert's resurrection and arrangement of William
Boyce's gay and graceful airs have put lovers of eighteenth-century
music eternally in his debt, and Roger Furse's Rowlandsonesque *décor*
includes a drop curtain with a Rabelaisian display of fine gauge,
fully fashioned silk stockings. At the sight of this in war-time the
heart of the feminine portion of the audience broke with an audible
crack.

ORPHEUS AND EURYDICE : PROMENADE

NINETTE DE VALOIS'S only other serious and large-scale
work during the war, *Orpheus and Eurydice*, produced at the New
Theatre in 1941, disappeared from the repertoire in 1942, although
this original experiment in the use of dance and mime as illustration
of a vocal score, harking back to the use of singers in the Diaghileff–
Nijinska–Stravinsky ballet *Les Noces*, was of sufficient interest and
success to warrant revival. Gluck's music for the characters of Orpheus
and Eurydice was sung offstage as an accompaniment to the action;
the ballet took on, as a result, the character of a danced opera and the
only disparity and awkwardness were due to an inherent difficulty in
this particular score, the male part in Gluck's opera being scored for
a contralto voice which proceeded rather oddly from the person of
Robert Helpmann, miming the part of Orpheus. The sustained sweep
and grandeur of this music was beautifully matched by the choreographer in the mourning movements and grouping of the opening
scene, the funeral of Eurydice, an exquisite study in black and white

Grecian classicism by Sophie Fedorovich, and the scene in Hades had some choreographic power accentuated by a fine piece of staging in which monumental shadows of the dancing groups were thrown in triplicate on the backcloth.

The return to the world was marked by some dances for children and lovers which had the freshness of spring flowers after rain, and in the part of one of the lovers, created by John Hart and June Brae, a youthful dancer of copper-haired beauty and shining grace, Moira Shearer, later made her first radiant appearance outside the *corps de ballet* in this company. For the first time, also, the choreographer created a part for Margot Fonteyn—the grave and delicately understanding figure of Love who leads the stricken Orpheus to the underworld in search of his dead Eurydice—which was entirely suited to her, and the aching sense of bereavement in this loveliest and, at the last, most tragic of all love stories was never lost in this ballet, the part of the restored Eurydice being beautifully conceived and played both by its creator, Pamela May, and her successor Julia Farron. Orpheus was a study in stylised mime rather lacking in variety: Helpmann's success in it could only be gauged when it was afterwards played by another dancer who had not the sensitive personality of the artist-musician nor the same expressive control of gesture.

The London *première* of Ninette de Valois's last war-time ballet, *Promenade*, on 7th December 1943, was notable for the unusual event of the company's *prima ballerina*, Margot Fonteyn, appearing as understudy at short notice for a younger dancer, Beryl Grey, in addition to several other last-minute changes of cast. A ballet suffering from an attack of influenza is, like a woman, not normally seen at its best; and it says much for the resilience of the Sadler's Wells company that in this case the exception proved the rule. The distinctive elements of this ballet are spontaneity and "style," the last an elusive quality but one that can give to a small light work of this nature an elegance that does not fade when the first novelty is past. In another sense also *Promenade* is a pattern of *divertissement* ballet construction; it has the connecting link between the dances, and the sustained atmosphere, that distinguish true choreography from the mere arrangement of dances, and make even so slight a work a ballet complete and coherent in itself.

The scene of the ballet is a park, for which the designer, Hugh Stevenson, has conceived a stylised setting in autumnal green and burnt sienna, and sparse trees that bend in naked beauty of line above the silken prettiness of French Empire costumes. The connecting link between the dances is provided by an elderly lepidopterist, whose exits and entrances, book-engrossed or in pursuit of an evasive butterfly, have the humour of the unexpected, suddenly turning a *pas de trois* into a *pas de quatre* and relieving the *longueurs* of the least inventive dance in the ballet, into which his flying appearance has the surprise value of a chord in Haydn's Symphony No. 94 in G. Gordon Hamilton achieved in this part an admirable small character study in which benevolent abstraction and little ripples of vexation were amusingly blended, and it is difficult to imagine the ballet without him.

A romantic *pas de deux*, danced on the first night by Margot Fonteyn with David Paltenghi as a strikingly handsome and sympathetic partner, contains some grave, swinging "lifts" and an attractive use of *battements cloches*, and its faint, bitter-sweet nostalgia of farewell was echoed in Margot Fonteyn's performance, which had something of the autumnal wistfulness of her forsaken Flower Girl in *Nocturne*. It has been charmingly danced since—though never again quite so tenderly—by Moira Shearer, Pamela May and Beryl Grey. Shearer's crystalline precision and vivacity, a new aspect of this dancer's work, were sparklingly apparent in the *pas de trois*, an original combination of one character and two classical dancers in which Ray Powell and Alexis Rassine also shone, and the ballet's one solo proved an equally witty study in *gaminerie*. This solo of a youthful minx, bored and bent on mischief, was excellently danced by Pauline Clayden, who brought to the nut-brown little maid a shrugging petulance, cheekiness and delight at her ephemeral male "capture" that were wholly enchanting. The elaborate figurations of a very fine Breton folk dance, in the arrangement of which Miss de Valois was assisted by Lieutenant de Cadenet of the Fighting French Air Force, bring the ballet to a spirited and breathless conclusion, and the dancing rhythms of Haydn's music are gaily reflected throughout. This ballet, like Miss de Valois's stylish Watteau-Handel *pastorale*, *The Gods Go A-Begging*, is one of those slight works which to retain their freshness require a high degree of expertness in characterisation and technique; when it receives this *Promenade* makes a bright and piquant opening to a programme, and there is room for such in all ballet repertoires.

The all-absorbing and arduous duties of directorship in war-time have prevented Ninette de Valois from exercising to the full her gifts as a major choreographer, and *Checkmate*, her most intricate and, after *The Rake's Progress* and *Job*, most powerfully dramatic ballet, first performed at the Paris Exhibition, was not revived after the production was lost in Holland. A work such as *Promenade* can, in a choreographer of such stature, only be a stopgap, and with her brain and graphic grasp of character, her total lack of sentimentality, her sense of dramatic detail and virility in the conception of male and chorus dances, Ninette de Valois may yet discover new paths for English ballet.

CHAPTER XII

FREDERICK ASHTON AND SADLER'S WELLS

JUDGED from any point of view and by any standards, the ballets of Frederick Ashton have been a potent force in the development of English ballet, and in quality of dance and imagination they compare in most cases with the work of the greatest choreographers of any other country. Ashton is the poet of English ballet, basing his ballets far more than Ninette de Valois on variety and invention in the use of classical dance steps, and at his best translating pure movement and plastic line into an abstract plane of lyric beauty and sensitivity to pain. Ashton's early training with Massine and experience in the company of Ida Rubinstein, in addition to his natural artistic instinct, have given him a cosmopolitan style in composition which makes his ballets more conceivable as a part of a foreign company's repertoire than those of any other English choreographer; he is less subject to outside influences of literature and art, and though always expressive and often dramatic his work is objective rather than subjective in theme and feeling. He has always had remarkable facility, but his work has increased steadily in character and spiritual depth, and both the fashionable slickness and buoyant humour of some of his earlier ballets have disappeared in his later works. It is as if the outpouring of pent-up emotion in his masterpiece, *Dante Sonata*, in 1940, had drained his spirit of sparkle and frivolity, and in his following work of relaxation, *The Wise Virgins*, the fun is only incidental and entirely subordinate to a new grace and serenity of spirit. Ashton as an artist has now reached complete maturity; but the blithe inconsequence of his lighter ballets was never crass, and they continue to give invaluable balance to the Sadler's Wells repertoire.

FAÇADE : LES RENDEZVOUS : LES PATINEURS

FAÇADE, originally produced for the Camargo Society, is the earliest of Ashton's ballets to have retained a permanent place in

Sadler's Wells programmes, and although an unmistakable child of its period, the fashionable sophisticated satire of the late nineteen-twenties and early nineteen-thirties, its wit and classical burlesque, together with William Walton's music, have saved it from staleness. The original *décor* of John Armstrong, nonsensically suggestive but stylish, fitted the spirit of the ballet in a way the Edwardian music hall vulgarity of the same artist's later setting has failed to do, and the dance of the Milkmaid and her swains has, since redressing, entirely lost its Tyrolese flavour. For this reason the performances given by the Ballet Rambert with the original *décor* and costumes, though less good in respect of individual dancing, are to-day more satisfying as a reproduction of Ashton's original conception than those given by the Sadler's Wells company.

The style of this ballet, though there have been some good individual performances, tends to escape younger dancers, and since the war the ballet has pivoted more and more around Robert Helpmann's Dago. Ashton's original performance of this part, the satire of a true Latin American with that instinctive Spanish heritage of "style" he recognises and admires in the people of his birthplace, has been changed by Helpmann into a burlesque of a pseudo-Latin gigolo of the type that during the tango period haunted the dancing salons of the north. It bears as much relation to the original as the society tango watched ironically by that pure *hidalgo* in spirit, R. B. Cunninghame Graham, in Paris bore to the fierce and passionate dance he had seen performed, with murder in its train, in his early days among the gauchos of South America. But in comedy spontaneity and invention are of infinitely more value than a painstaking imitation of a previous interpretation; the riot of your true comedian can never be suppressed, and Helpmann's disreputable and "phony" Dago, overglossed and beringed, flashing of eye, wickedly undulating of hand and foot, is a piece of slippery innuendo that fits easily into the ballet and has done its share in lightening the burdens of war.

In *Rendezvous*, the first ballet created by Ashton for Sadler's Wells, satire is softened to a gay light humour and for the first time his mastery of classical movement becomes apparent. This is classical dancing very nearly for its own sake, but with a thread of idea—a series of variations on the American theme of Boy Meets Girl—that runs through the whole ballet and is sustained with infinite variety and charm. *Rendezvous* has everything a light vehicle for pure dancing should have: pattern and fluid beauty of line, precision and high spirits, dances for soloists and corps which exploit technique with an eye for grouping and balance as well as virtuosity of movement. It contains a *pas de trois* of unique sauciness and *ballon* which was danced originally by Ninette de Valois, Stanley Judson and Robert Helpmann and in which Margaret Dale and Joan Sheldon have more recently displayed particular sparkle and poise. And although the velocity and flame-like, quivering mobility of Idzikowsky and Markova—those qualities that made their Blue Birds memorable—were entirely their own, Robert Helpmann, John Hart and Alexis Rassine have in war-time danced the male solo with attractive fluency, and Margot Fonteyn and the youthful Beryl Grey—less balanced and elegant but fresh and volatile as a spring breeze—have succeeded Markova with individual charm. Auber's music gives this ballet the effervescence of champagne; but this alcoholic stimulation unfortunately proved too much for the inexperienced legs of the war-time male corps, and in their performance of the *pas de six*, a difficult study in clean classical execution, this ballet met its temporary Waterloo.

Much the same fate has in recent years attended *Les Patineurs*. This ballet, like *Les Rendezvous*, is an outstanding example of how a work with a very slight theme—in this case merely a vividly sustained atmosphere of the skating rink—may retain permanent interest through the sheer scintillating variety of its dance invention. *Les Patineurs* is a display of technical fireworks without a damp squib, and the cross-currents of its patterns have a flowing charm. But if its technicalities are to seem part of the general picture and not a series of virtuoso feats they must be performed by the dancers with the maximum of effortlessness and joy of movement. The freedom and spontaneity of Mary Honer's *fouettés*, Harold Turner's arrow-like swiftness, the lyrical splendour given to the figures of the two skaters in white by Robert Helpmann and Margot Fonteyn as they wove a strand of poetry and romance through the bright spinning tapestry of the other skaters—these have created a precedent which will only be equalled as a whole when this ballet is once again treated as a principal work in which the "star" dancers of the company are not considered too important to appear. The return of Pamela May, partnered beautifully by Beryl Grey, showed the truth of this, and the white skimming radiance of Moira Shearer in the *pas de deux* has recaptured the same feeling of absolute quality. At Covent Garden also the young dancer Avril Navarre has given to the *fouettés* a renewed speed and assurance. The frosty crispness of William Chappell's designs and Meyerbeer's tunes provide a gay framework for this ballet, which is choreo-graphically equal to anything in a like genre produced by Russian companies.

THE WEDDING BOUQUET

IN' *The Wedding Bouquet*, Ashton's major comic work, his humour once again becomes directed into channels of classical dance satire, but with a maturity of idea and rich crazy variety of movement far in advance of the chic parody of *Façade*. Sophistication is the quality in which English ballet is most generally lacking, and it is this which gives to the *pastiche* of *The Wedding Bouquet* its original and pungent flavour. This Lord Berners–Frederick Ashton ballet is therefore of value, not only in itself, but in giving "tone" to the Sadler's Wells repertoire as a whole. The peculiar daftness of Gertrude Stein's verses, originally sung but now spoken as an accompaniment, is matched by Lord Berners's witty play with ragtime rhythms and Edwardian costumes, as well as Ashton's tongue-in-the-cheek varia-tions on classical *pas*, and the whole has an inspired idiocy that blows through the theatre with the gusty exhilaration of a March wind.

Ashton's dance invention is throughout astonishing, and his amusing variety of "lifts" and exits leaves one breathless. The first entrance of the Bridegroom magnificently blends surprise and absurdity, and only a master choreographer could have devised this ballet's burlesque of the classical *pas de deux*, in which even the music achieves a malicious parody of the *Casse Noisette* type of *Adagio*, with its elaborate preparation and climax. In the revival of this ballet in 1943 it was danced with beautiful mock-solemnity by Robert Helpmann and Margaret Dale, who has proved an admirable successor to Mary Honer as the Bride, quivering of eyelash, vacant in charm, and with the firm dancing line and attack of a miniature ballerina. Her well-bred oblivion to the intrusion of her groom's purple past is one of the delights of the ballet, and she is French to her fingertips. Helpmann's Bridegroom, harassed by fainting Bride, clinging ex-flame and all the ghastly social ritual that civilisation inflicts on those about to wed, remains, if hardly a thing of beauty, at least a joy for ever, and wears a dotty moustache and centre parting to the manner born. Helpmann has all the *nuances* of burlesque at his fingertips and his pre-ballet experience in musical comedy and revue enables him to carry off a Burlington Bertie skit quite outside the range of the average dancer. His one fault, as a comedian, is a sense of fun so strong that he occasionally loses control of it and laughs at himself. Margot Fonteyn manages to be at once haywire and forlorn as the local Mad Margaret or Petite Fadette, a part requiring considerable technique as well as a lunatically unmanageable coiffure. To play Giselle one night and Julia in this ballet the next requires an extremely sensitive adjustment of balance which Fonteyn has now attained to a nicety. Of the rest, Grace Greenway in the revival proved a little dog with taking ways and neat ballerina's points, Moyra Fraser's Josephine had tipsy Edwardian archness and Alexis Rassine, in a burgundy blouse and remarkably ill-fitting cream flannels, performed some elastic and irrelevant gyrations of which no one on the stage appeared to dream of taking any notice whatsoever. Lord Berners's photographic décor (of Lake Kammer, Salzkammergut, Austria) is charmingly effective and Constant Lambert, reading the Stein verses from the dignified detachment of the New Theatre Royal Box, inimitably gave point to the pointless.

This use of nonsensical spoken verse as an accompaniment to movement was at the time of the creation of *The Wedding Bouquet* a new departure in ballet; it requires expert wit and timing in the accompanying action but when it has this the result can be extraordinarily funny. Frank Staff later created his funniest scene in *Peter and the Wolf*, that of the Huntsmen, to the spoken narrative that occurs in Prokofiev's score, but in stark craziness *The Wedding Bouquet* stands alone, nonsense vitalised by wit and still the most unique of Ashton's ballets.

APPARITIONS : THE WISE VIRGINS

APPARITIONS was Ashton's first work on a dramatic scale, one in which his romanticism, poetry and sense of lurking and indefinable tragedy first became apparent and through which the nature and depth of his genius could be fairly gauged. For *Apparitions*, based like Massine's ballet on Berlioz's dramatic programme of the *Symphonie Fantastique*, is an evocation of romanticism as complete as that of Fokine in *Sylphides*, though it deals with a totally different angle of the movement. With its atmosphere of dream and nightmare, its Byronic drugtaking poet and vision of an ideal Beloved, its tolling bells and Devil's Cavern, this ballet captures that spirit of macabre fantasy that haunted Shelley and Mary Godwin in the stories of Monk Lewis, that gave birth to *Frankenstein* and invaded the work of Byron and the romantic poets. Yet Ashton has miraculously avoided melodrama, and touched the whole scene with a burning and tender imagination.

In every revival the ballet has retained its power to move and its crescendo of mounting excitement. The beautiful gradation of colour in Cecil Beaton's costumes, and Constant Lambert's fine arrangement of Liszt's music, combine with the richness and invention of the dance to suggest an atmosphere at once vivid and yet touched with the sinister imprint of a dream. This emphasis on the unreal is enhanced by Robert Helpmann's acting as the Poet, especially in the magnificent Ball Scene when he seems to move in another dimension, with the dancers and yet not of them. Helpmann dances this exhausting part with fire and passionate sincerity, and his grief in the funeral scene, his sense of the fugitive, and the shock of disillusion in his face as the Beloved slips from his embrace into the arms of the Hussar, are among his most moving achievements. Margot Fonteyn beautifully realises the dream-like fascination, half-tender, half-capricious, of the Woman in the Ball Dress, and like Helpmann she has still in this ballet one of her greatest parts.

Apparitions was rarely revived in war-time and the smallness of the New Theatre stage did not enable its mobile and exciting pattern to be seen at its best. In its brief appearances in the repertoire it has provided an interesting contrast to Ashton's later, less ambitious but delicately complete exercise in dramatic narration, *The Wise Virgins*. In this ballet Ashton, without attempting any metaphysical or psychological suggestion, has translated the Bach music into a series of dissolving pictures of Renaissance beauty, telling his story with the simplicity of an illustrated fairy tale and most sensitively echoing the composer's serene, firm texture in the hand movements of the Bride and the charming flexible groupings of the Cherubs. Prince Peter Lieven in his intelligent and thoughtful book, *The Birth of the Ballets-Russe*, expressed the view that the abstract music of Bach could never be matched on the stage except in completely abstract movement: *The Wise Virgins* shows the only other balletic possibility, the expression of the religious feeling of certain of Bach's music through the symbolic pictures of a Bible parable. The whole ballet has a sweeping fluidity of progression and its flaws are due, perhaps, more to performance than conception, the sustained poses of the angels never being achieved with sufficient balance for the static grouping to make its full pictorial effect. The Bridegroom, too, is a figure of stylised benevolence extremely difficult to mime convincingly, and the costumes of the male dancers are not helpful. Yet with Rex Whistler's pellucid Italianate colour and rococo setting this ballet has the beauty, at times, of an old master, and the exquisitely conceived character of the Bride becomes, in Margot Fonteyn's hands, the pivot of the ballet, a figure of fresco-like innocence and grace. The frivolity of the Foolish Virgins darts across the limpid surface of the ballet like a shaft of sunlight, and Mary Honer as their leader plumbed depths of disarming silliness no one has ever achieved since.

DANTE SONATA : THE WANDERER

ASHTON'S instinct has always been towards abstraction rather than narrative, and the creation not of realistic characters but of symbols of humanity expressed through beauty of movement, pattern and "line". His is the painter's eye rather than the dramatist's: "Action in ballet," he has written to me in a letter, "should (in my opinion) be choreographic and tense and not solely theatric, for when it is only theatric and steps into the world of drama one feels the lack of the spoken word. Dramatic action should be translated into the choreographic idea." Certainly this personal outlook is apparent in all Ashton's work, and it is the replacement of poetry of language by poetry of movement that has become the essence of his ideal as an artist, the waking dream which in his greatest ballets he has striven again and again to realise, and rarely without success. *Horoscope*, his first serious large-scale exercise in abstraction, in which the dramatic and the lyrical were expressed through a purely plastic arrangement of design, marked an inevitable phase in his development, and anticipated the heightened spiritual suggestion of *Dante Sonata* and *The Wanderer* later.

Of these three abstract ballets only *Dante Sonata*, to the music of Liszt, has remained continuously in the repertoire, an expression of human suffering and conflict that has extraordinary power and anguish. It is the product of extreme emotional stress, the overflow of personal tragedy and spiritual unrest as well as of the larger issues of war and the forces of evil. A great deal has been read into this ballet that the choreographer never intended to put there, and only at one graphic moment, when the Children of Darkness tramp and surge over the helpless bodies of their victims on the ground, is it directly inspired by the tragedy of Nazi-invaded Poland; but the very inexplicitness of its despair gives it a sharper poignancy, it is like that chilling cry of revelation and protest that rends the fabric of the last scene of *Juno and the Paycock*, "There isn't a God, there isn't a God"! In a *finale* of bitter potency the Children of Light are crucified beside the Children of Darkness: only the central figure, transfigured in light, expresses the possibility of hope for humanity and the world.

Choreographically Ashton has proved equal to his theme and music; his fluctuating patterns and rushing lines have strength and complexity and excitement; the vicious abandon of evil is suggested in sensuous bodies and an entanglement of arms and legs against which a girl, half-submerged, fights with a drowning desperation; a hand uplifted or covering a face has a terrible suggestiveness; two mourners follow a bier in a pose eloquent of grief and behind them a woman of darkness with trembling hands, crouched to spring, fills the empty stage after their departure with a sense of nameless terror. The tragic impact of *Dante Sonata* is such that when it was performed in Holland just before the Nazi invasion the Dutch audience rose in their seats and cheered the company. It has been consistently well performed by a changing team of Sadler's Wells dancers, among whom Margot Fonteyn has remained memorable in musical expressiveness and emotional intensity. Robert Helpmann, June Brae and Celia Franca have led the Children of Darkness with baleful dæmonism, and at Covent Garden Beryl Grey has danced the leading figure of evil with a plastic power of movement of extraordinary ferocity and eloquence. Pamela May has also given a fine emotional balance to the work, her frenzied pain and resignation matching the moving performance of Margot Fonteyn. Constant Lambert's arrangement of the Liszt sonata for piano and orchestra has intensified its drama, and here as in *Nocturne* and *Horoscope*, lost in Holland in 1940, Ashton is indebted to Sophie Fedorovitch for *décor* and costumes, inspired by Flaxman, that imaginatively realise the movement and atmosphere.

Dante Sonata exploits to the utmost the sinuosity of the human body, its power to express feeling, in free dance movement of compelling variety. With *The Wanderer*, a year later, Ashton returned to the framework of classical technique, which he here used with an invention, intricacy and sense of the spectacular in movement which he had never before attained. *The Wanderer* is a new and mentally stimulating development in ballet, a combination of electric brilliance of technique with a sense of spiritual growth through experience. Massine's symphonic ballets, in which the characters are dream figures or symbols of life and destiny, never attempted to touch the deeper problems of human psychology, but the nostalgia of the Schubert song which Liszt transcribed for piano and orchestra has given Ashton a more personal scope of theme which he has illustrated with profound compassion and insight. For the Wanderer of this ballet is a wanderer in the Byronic sense, a representation of man in his earthly pleasure, suffering and spiritual renascence. *Dante Sonata* is the tragedy of all humanity; *The Wanderer* the tragedy and the triumph of the individual soul.

The three phases of this spiritual progression act as a deeply sensitive expression of the three movements of the music; as a result the ballet is an artistically welded unity of music, choreography and idea in which the glittering allure of life in the first scene and the Wanderer's conquering of disillusion and pain in the last are paralleled in movement of thrilling acrobacy and impetuosity, and linked by an *adagio* in which the flexibility of the grouping and the dragging of the Wanderer's body in the dust seem like an intensification of Shelley's tortured cry, "I fall upon the thorns of life! I bleed!"

The technical virtuosity is throughout remarkable; it blinds like the flash of a diamond in the sun. The figure of the Wanderer is lifted on the crest of groups that surge upwards like the tidal wave of Hokusai's print, break and re-form into new architectural patterns and lines; the woman who is the embodiment of worldly allure, danced by Margot Fonteyn with a magnificent and tingling vitality that showed a completely new facet of her art, is tossed to the Wanderer, caught and spun in midair, sent in one sweeping movement down the full length of his body, head foremost, to the ground; two women pirouette in a circle into which the Wanderer and a third woman are drawn in a sudden whirling ecstasy of physical excitement. And always the athleticism is punctuated with passages of tranquil immobility and grace. Two young lovers enter in a caressing *pas de deux* of pastel lyricism; the compassionate figure of a woman searches for the Wanderer in the tragic second movement, lifts and comforts him like a bruised child in his agony; two young children dance across the scene like heralds of spring, dream figments in the teeming and pain-haunted imagination of the Wanderer. All these parts were sensitively played in the first performances by Pamela May and Michael Somes, Julia Farron, and the youthful Margaret Dale and Deryk Mendel, and the entrance of the children was marked by Robert Helpmann with a facial expression of strange pathos, one of those rare and indefinable moments in performance that touch both heart and imagination and remain imprinted on the memory. Helpmann danced and mimed the central figure throughout with a concentrated beauty and poignancy of expression and revealed here in a more intense form than ever before that power, which he shares with Massine, of riveting the attention even in immobility and making the other dancers seem an emanation of his mind. The costumes were not uniformly successful (though entirely so in the case of the Wanderer himself) but Graham Sutherland's glowing backcloths beautifully accentuated the living and flexible line of the choreography.

THE QUEST

THE WANDERER, a refutation of Gautier's theory that ballet is powerless to suggest the metaphysical and an important new development in choreographic expression, was the last ballet produced by Ashton before he volunteered for the Forces in 1941. *The Quest*, produced at the New Theatre on 6th April 1943 during a temporary leave of absence from the R.A.F., is the only other ballet he was able to create in war-time. Though a less homogeneous work than *Dante Sonata* and *The Wanderer*, *The Quest*, based on Book I of Spenser's *Faerie Queene* and a return to the narrative form of ballet, once again revealed Ashton as a master mind of ballet, one with an exceptional grasp of technical resources and understanding of his dancers. The work was given an added distinction through the collaboration of two other artists, William Walton and John Piper, outstanding in their particular spheres. Walton's music, with its dramatic impact, atmosphere and force and ingenuity of rhythm, is an important contribution to the ballet and John Piper's *décor* shows at its best a picturesque feeling for the romantic tradition, his mystic forest of the opening scene and costumes for Una and the Bats being particularly notable.

Spenser's allegory is the least successful element in the ballet; perhaps because Ashton is always happier with a theme than with a story. The action, in spite of its complications of disguise, is dramatic and not difficult to follow; but the kernel of Spenser's conception of St. George, a knight youthful and untested, is the spiritual growth of a character who, knowing the tearing inner conflict of temptation and disillusion, conquers both and finds in the House of Holinesse the healing purity and peace of mind without which he is still unfitted for his great quest to England. This aspect of the House of Holinesse is insufficiently clear in the ballet, the Red Cross Knight having long since appeared to be, like the heroine of *Measure for Measure*, "ensky'd and sainted." Choreographically, too, St. George lacks variety, this being the one part in which Ashton has failed to reveal to advantage the finest attribute of his dancer, Helpmann's magnificent "line." Helpmann is too sensitive and imaginative an artist not to give to the rôle more than he finds in it, and after a few performances in which he seemed still to be feeling his way he built the character into a dramatically consistent whole, touched by suffering and disillusion but with the still centre of integrity of the saint. With its sadness of spirit and sinewy litheness this performance realised exactly the Spenserian ideal of a knight errant.

The only other choreographic weakness in this production is in the use of the *corps de ballet* in the Palace of Pride, the lack of a strong male team having betrayed Ashton into the creation of a corps of hermaphrodites, a suggestion of viciousness that failed through inadequacy of make-up and performance. The dance here lacks the authority of Ashton's best work, and the costume design, smacking of popular revue, does not help. The dances of the Seven Deadly Sins are, however, cleverly arranged, notably so in the case of Avarice and the climax dance of Pride, the Queen, splendidly built around Moira Shearer's high arabesque and firmness of balance. This young dancer brought to the part a shining imperious beauty and self-absorption that marked her out as dancer and mime. Ashton's flair for drawing out the best in the dancer to illustrate the rôle was also apparent in his handling of Beryl Grey, then a fifteen-year-old child who had already danced the dual ballerina rôles in *Lac des Cygnes* and who gave to the false Duessa of this ballet a flashing vitality and sensuousness that showed a remarkable advance as an artist. Technically this is the most glittering part in the ballet, including some striking supported arabesque turns, rhythmic flexions of arms and wrists and one exit with St. George, the sword pointed treacherously at the knight's back, that is masterly.

The master's hand is, in fact, apparent from the first scene, which Ashton enriches with an atmosphere of wizardry unmatched since Fokine created Kostchei in *L'Oiseau de Feu*. Throughout the ballet there is a wealth of invention; in the quivering crossed hands and staccato pointwork of the Bats, excellently danced in the original production by Pauline Clayden and Lorna Mossford; the bizarrely imagined Wizard, Archimago, and his sycophant, to which Leslie

Edwards and Celia Franca gave a mimic vividness; the fights with the Saracens, excitingly conceived in terms of dance and with one fine climax when Sansjoy, played with dark savage strength by David Paltenghi, swings St. George in great wheeling circles off the ground; the serene mediæval grouping of the finale, with St. George in a red cloak that glows like the stained glass of a Cathedral window, and the tender *pas de deux* and farewell, with linked praying hands, that precedes it.

As in all Ashton's ballets the *pas de deux* are consistently excellent, and they range in mood from St. George's dance, half-fascinated, half-repelled, with the Wizard's temptress and Una's unsuspecting welcome of the disguised Archimago, with its sinister background of trumpet rhythms, to the shining happiness of her dance with the true St. George after his victory, when in a series of tiny "lifts" she seems to glide above the ground with winged feet. Margot Fonteyn and Robert Helpmann expressed in this dance a spring-like grace and lightness of heart, and Fonteyn's part of Una, the spirit of Truth, is a lyrical balletic expression of Spenser's golden verse. She has never danced with more tenderness and charm, and her slow walk across the stage with St. George, on beautifully arched points, is one of Ashton's happiest inventions.

There has been a sensitive and charming performance of Una since by Pauline Clayden, but both the parts of Duessa and Pride have proved difficult to recast and Helpmann's non-appearance has emphasised how much the character of St. George depended on his subtleties of expression and ability to give a danceable quality to a fairly static rôle. The right balance of physique between St. George and the Saracens, chivalry and spirit opposed to brute force, has also proved necessary to preserve the design of the dances and Spenser's moral. The folly of too extensive "doubling" of rôles has been more apparent here than in any of Ashton's ballets except *Les Patineurs*. He is, as he himself realises, intensively responsive to the dancers for whom he creates and it is only when they dance that a perfect contact with Ashton's conception is established and the subtleties of movement, which tend gradually to get lost when passed from hand to hand, are fully revealed. *The Quest* is not the greatest of Ashton's ballets but it is a work of considerable choreographic invention that in a good performance can be moving as well as exciting. In its alliance of three of the foremost contemporary minds in choreography, music and painting, it has real importance.

NOCTURNE

THE transfer of the Sadler's Wells Ballet from the New to the Princes Theatre, with its accommodation for a larger orchestra, made possible the revival, on 28th October 1944, of *Nocturne*, a ballet composed to the music of Delius's "Paris" Nocturne and dropped from the repertoire when the company was forced to leave Sadler's Wells Theatre in September 1940. Created in 1936, a short while after *Apparitions*, *Nocturne* was one of Ashton's earliest major works for the Wells, and it remains a masterly example of English ballet, a pure dance drama of flashing beauty in the Diaghileff tradition, with more continuity and compactness than *Apparitions* even though there is nothing in it, choreographically, to equal the matchless and dream-haunted Ball Scene of the earlier ballet, still Ashton's most poetic and sustained invention.

Historically, *Nocturne* is, perhaps, more important, since here for the first time Ashton composed to concert music more exacting than the essentially dramatic music of Liszt, and created a ballet with human characters set in a period not far distant from our own. The theme, suggested by Edward Sackville-West, a small human tragedy played out against a background of ball and masquerade in a great city by night, has been perfectly realised by the choreographer, who has set his four leading characters, the worldly young man, the rich girl he chooses, the poor girl he rejects, and the compassionate spectator who is moved from his detachment and lifts his arms over the city in a saddened philosophy, against shifting patterns of lifting and whirling dancers which break like waves over the three lovers, submerge, part and throw them together again. The dance moves upwards as well as forwards, the Rich Young Girl makes her entrance in a "lift" of winged ecstasy that carries her across the whole stage into the arms of her lover, a nameless girl kneels, with an impulsive gesture of sympathy, beside the weeping Flower Girl and the *corps de ballet* is established, not as a mere dancing background, but as a group of human characters.

The brief *pas de deux*, dances of swinging "lifts" and sensuous, intertwining arms, are finely inventive and expressive, and Ashton's opposition of masqueraders and ball dancers draws an effective choreographic parallel to the musical counterpoint. The nostalgic period atmosphere of Delius's score, with its bitter-sweet woodwind *motif* and sense of a great city sleeping and throbbing to life, the ballet beautifully realises in dance and design, Sophie Fedorovitch's costumes, flowing in line and warm in colour, being breathtakingly lovely, and the night sky and classic simplicity of her setting giving a curious sense of an invisible city below.

The chief weakness in this ballet was the solo of the Young Man, a meaningless dance which held up the action and did nothing to express his character or emotions. Its lack of virility may have been in part due to the music, whose sad melodic outline certainly does not call for male dancing at this moment, and the costume, evening dress and "tails," being more normally associated in dancing with revue and the music hall, is a difficult one for a solo in a serious ballet. Since this revival, however, the dance has been changed to include other dancers, with a consequent strengthening of the continuity of pattern.

The Flower Girl was one of the first parts created by Ashton for Margot Fonteyn, and with dances designed to reveal the charm of her arabesque and to express the mute pain of unrequited love it remains one of the most fragile and wistful of her portraits. The Rich Young Girl, created by the exotic and beautiful June Brae with sensational success, was played by Pamela May in the revival with a flushed radiance of youthful seductiveness and beauty, and Robert Helpmann, in a more sophisticated portrait than heretofore, did not minimise the purely sensual and selfish desire of the Young Man. Ashton himself, on leave from the R.A.F., returned to present a patrician profile to the audience and give the static rôle of the Spectator a positive value of pity and resignation which seemed to extend beyond the immediate action to all humanity in all time. The warmth of his reception showed the audience's awareness of how valuable an artist, as well as choreographer, ballet had lost during the past three and a half years.

How much English ballet has suffered in the creative sense by this prolonged inactivity of one of its greatest choreographers will never be truly estimated. Choreographers of talent are so rare and irreplaceable that the loss of one of them is infinitely more damaging than the loss of a playwright or actor to the theatre; nor is the effect on the artist's powers of invention likely to be anything but stultifying. "I believe artists should share, spiritually and physically, in the trials of their generation," Ashton has written; but while seeing the necessity and carrying it courageously into practice he has never blinded himself to the fact that inability to practise his art can lead only, in his belief, to sterility in the artist. Ashton has paid the price with his eyes wide open that lesser artists, developing their creative gifts and reputation during the war in another country, have not had to pay. Yet in the long run the harvest may be richer than the artist himself, feeling the chains of artistic inactivity, may realise. For Ashton's work is marked by mind as well as matter; *Dante Sonata* showed him acutely impressionable to external as well as personal emotion, and one of the ballets that has not ceased to foment in his restless imagination during the last years of the war may have a heightened psychological insight through his own frustration.

SYMPHONIC VARIATIONS

Symphonic Variations, produced at Covent Garden on 24th April 1946, and Ashton's first creative work since his release from the Forces, is not, however, a ballet of this nature. Perhaps partly as a reaction against the direction given to choreography by Robert Helpmann, with whose method of composition Ashton has by temperament little sympathy, and partly through some inner need, after so long an absence, to concentrate on the basis of ballet, the technique of the dance, Ashton in this work has stripped ballet free of all its accumulations of drama, emotion and stage production and produced his first purely abstract study in classical dance technique. In this he follows the line taken by Massine in *Choreartium*, also an attempt to parallel symphonic or "absolute" music in terms of "absolute" dance, although the Massine ballet, composed to the Fourth Symphony of Brahms, used an infinitely more complex form of choreography, including a good deal of architectural construction and grouping of dancers in the mass. Ashton, designing movement to a much lighter orchestral score—the Symphonic Variations for Piano and Orchestra by César Franck—has pared down his choreography to its barest simplicity and, composing for six soloists only without *corps de ballet*, devised what is, in essence, a long series of *enchaînements* for a few individual dancers who occasionally merge into a weaving line or small group but on the whole stand out singly or in pairs.

The question of the legitimacy of using symphonic music for choreographic purposes has been much debated in the past: certainly Massine's most successful ballet of this kind was the brilliant and beautiful *Symphonie Fantastique*, where he was able to use as his dramatic basis the imaginative narrative the composer himself had sought to express in music. But Berlioz's *Symphonie Fantastique* for this very reason does not quite fall into the category of "absolute" music, any more than do such concert works as Liszt's *Sonata Après une Lecture de Dante* (orchestrated by Constant Lambert) and Delius's "Paris" Nocturne, to which Ashton has previously composed successful ballets. The Schubert–Liszt fantasia *The Wanderer*, the second movement of which was a free transcription (first by Schubert for the piano, later by Liszt for piano and orchestra) of a Schubert song, also has a certain dramatic feeling and although Ashton translated the physical wanderer of the song, and his longing for his homeland, into a wanderer through life itself whose suffering was of a less definitive kind, at least the emotional mood of the music was fully sustained in the dance; indeed by accentuating its feeling the ballet added something, to my mind, to the music in a way a parallel of purely geometric dance patterns and technique cannot achieve.

But such an emotional translation does demand unusual sensitivity and taste on the part of the choreographer, and Massine's more obviously theatrical insertion of such figures as Fate, Frivolity and Anxiety into *Les Présages* seemed to me to diminish, rather than add to, the nobility of Tchaikovsky's music. Similarly his setting of a scene of Sodom and Gomorrah destruction to one of the happiest symphonic movements Beethoven ever composed prevented his *Seventh Symphony* from attaining any real artistic unity, in spite of the mourning Hebraic beauty of Bérard's crimson second movement, where for a brief space music, action and design became perfectly correlated in mood.

Unlike *Dante Sonata* and *The Wanderer*, I do not believe *Symphonic Variations* greatly heightens the impression of the music; but neither does it detract from it, and within its limitations the parallel of dance to music is sensitively sustained. There is no emotion in this dance beyond the lightest indication of grave or gay; the general impression, cool and serene, is enhanced by the soft green abstraction of Sophie Fedorovitch's backcloth, against which the dancers, in costumes whose simple Grecian lines exquisitely reveal the movements of the dance, shine white like daisies on a summer lawn. The costumes for two of the men, with bared shoulder and a single ring of black against the white, are superb. This is the perfection of ballet designing, and Ashton's debt to the artist is a great one.

Perhaps the principal value of the choreography lies in the fact that although the dance is purely technical, and owing to the length of the music extremely exhausting to the dancers, the technicalities

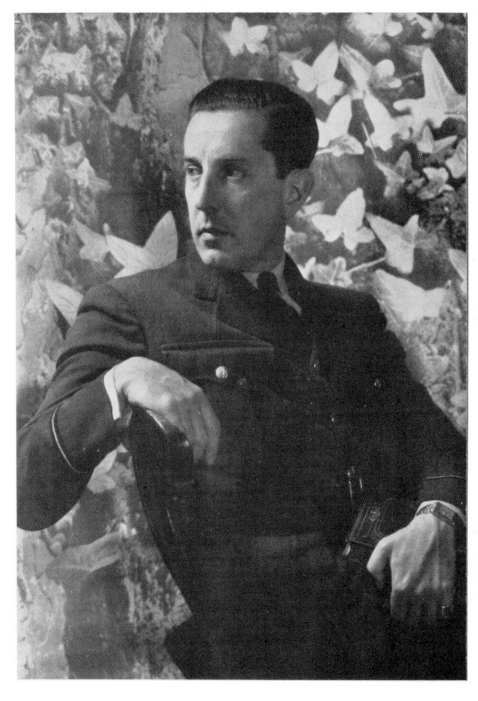

Photo

Frederick Ashton.

Cecil Beaton

Plate XXI

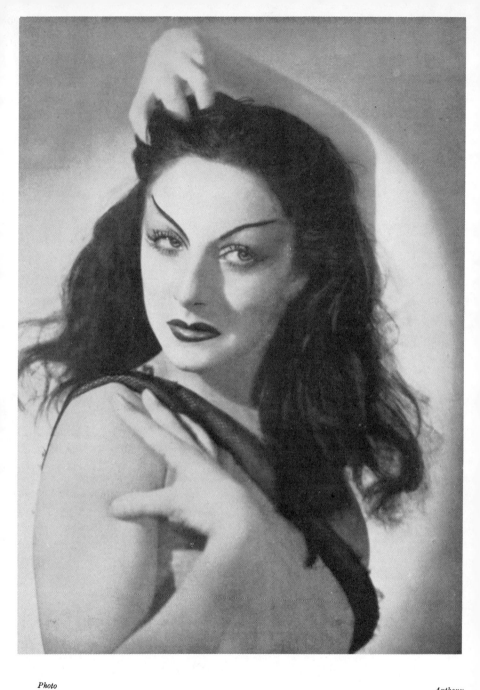

Photo

Anthony

Dante Sonata
Study in evil: Celia Franca

Plate XXII

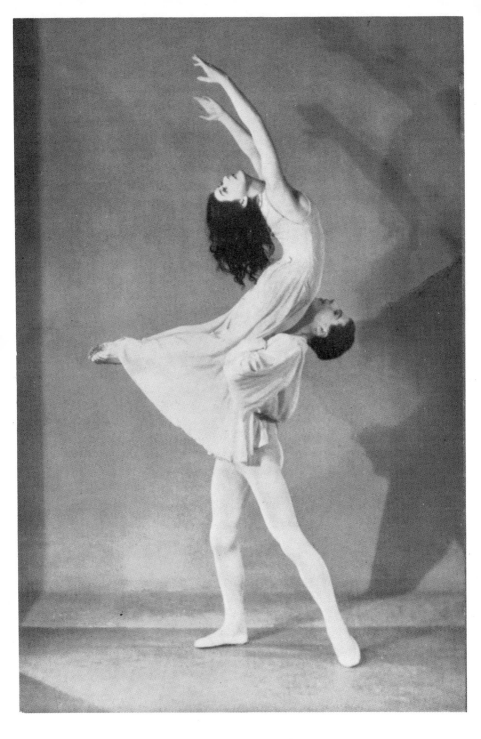

Dante Sonata
Children of Light: Margot Fonteyn and Michael Somes

Plate XXIII

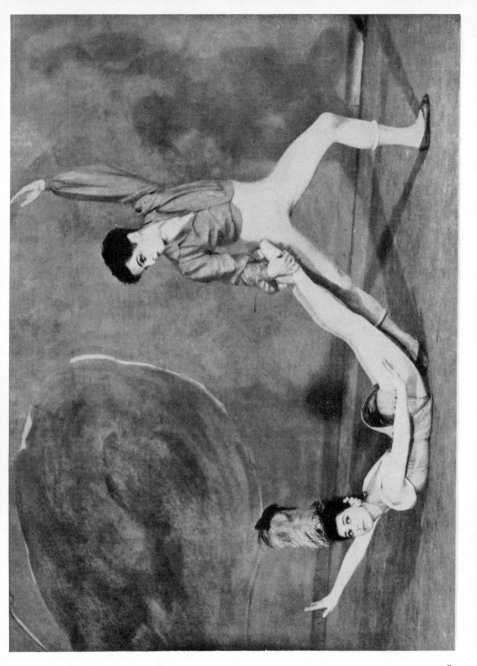

The Wanderer: Arrested Movement: Margot Fonteyn and Robert Helpmann.

Plate XXIV

Photo   W. Debenham

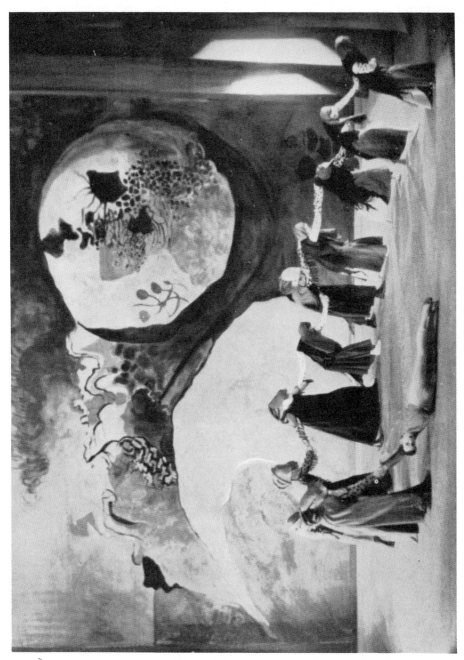

Plate XXV

The Wanderer: Second Movement (*Adagio*). *Décor* by Graham Sutherland.

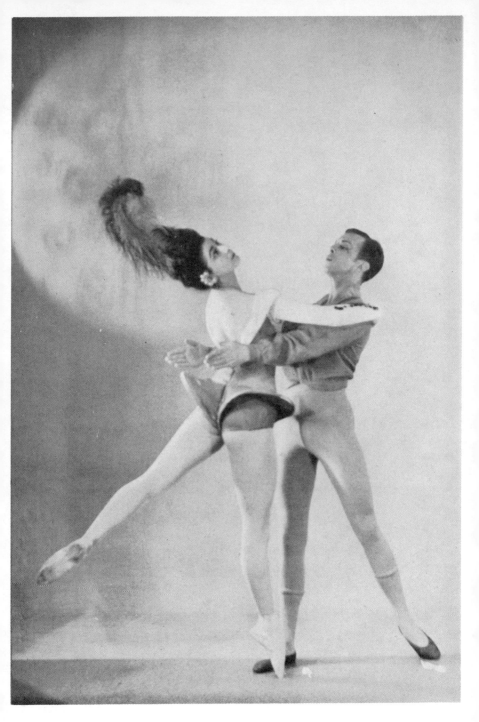

The Wanderer
Margot Fonteyn and Robert Helpmann

Plate XXVI

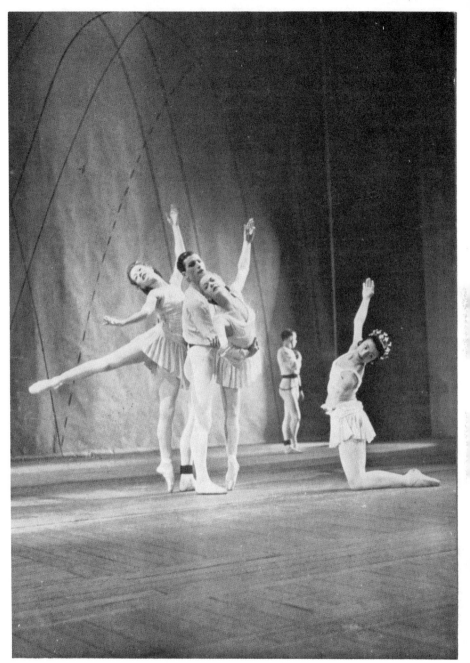

Symphonic Variations
Moira Shearer, Michael Somes, Pamela May, Brian Shaw and Margot Fonteyn.
Plate XXVII

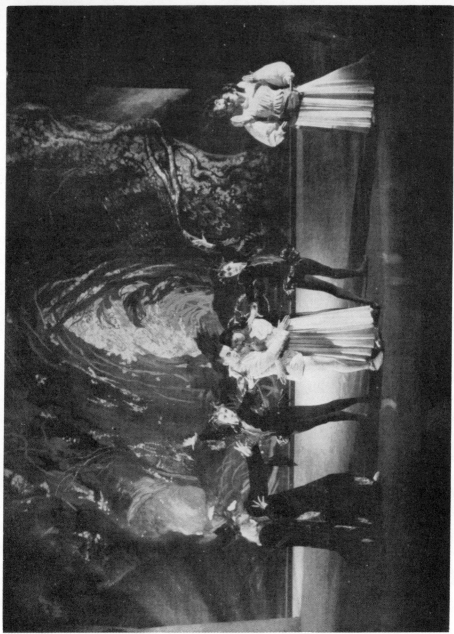

The Quest:
First Scene.
Décor by John
Piper.

Plate XXVIII

Photo *Tunbridge-Sedgwick*

never obtrude as such; the movement seems fluent, easy, unhurried, and though not without strength (notably in the noble and eloquent variation designed for Brian Shaw) it is invariably graceful. If the reduction of ballet to pure dance mathematics is in itself something of a retrogression, this technical achievement seems to me undoubtedly a progressive step in Ashton's mastery of dance movement. He is now in such complete command of his materials that one is unconscious of difficulties and the formalised style of the classic technique seems to spring from the most natural physical reactions. In this one sees his maturity and experience in comparison with the young French choreographers of *Les Ballets des Champs-Élysées*, seen in England at the time this ballet was produced. There the dance invention was also considerable, but it frequently underlined the acrobacy and showed a certain awkwardness, a lack of ease, in the taking up or changing of positions and groups.

The dance in *Symphonic Variations* is never spectacular but it is fresh and attractive to the eye; there are several charming "lifts," three girls in attitude wrap themselves like a white cloud round the central male figure, two of them cut diagonally across the stage in a gay little sequence of *échappés*, the men move forward in proud and sculptured *attitudes*, the girls pirouette round the men with a curious upward spiral movement of the arm. The line and rhythm of the music are reflected in hands and arms as well as feet, and although the brief *pas de deux*, danced by Margot Fonteyn and Michael Somes, is evocative—Ashton has used a similar succession of floating "lifts" in the *pas de deux* of both *The Wanderer* and *The Quest*—its lightness has an undying charm.[1]

A more serious criticism is the repetition of movement which occurs in all parts Ashton has built around Michael Somes; the dancer's technical limitations at the time of this ballet's production and the revival of *The Sleeping Beauty*, in which he danced Florestan, were partly attributable to a knee injury as well as his long service in the Armed Forces, but there is no doubt they have weakened English male choreography in variety and scope. Nevertheless he partnered in this ballet very well, and his subtle and instinctive musical phrasing is always valuable in a work of this kind. The other

[1] The repertoire of dance technique is, of course, even to-day not limitless and all choreographers at some time will echo, almost unconsciously, previous works by themselves or others. The same is true of writers and poets, with a far greater vocabulary at their disposal. It is only when it happens regularly that one can blame the artist.

two men, Henry Danton and Brian Shaw, were both creating their first leading part for this company. Danton's rôle extended little beyond supporting work, but his lightness, ease and purity of "line" were in the *danseur noble* tradition of style. Brian Shaw, a seventeen-year-old, had already shown virtuosity as the Blue Skater in *Les Patineurs* and in his solo here he displayed a virility, grace and control that marked him as the most promising young male dancer English ballet had produced for some years. He, also, has a fine, fluid "line"; his principal need in this ballet was for more vitality of expression.

The most difficult dancing fell to Margot Fonteyn, Moira Shearer and Pamela May, the company's three Auroras who displayed notable classical style and were in physique and colouring—ebony, auburn and gold—excellently matched. The continuation of the music, which, not being composed for dance, allows the dancers or choreographers no rest, causes a certain flagging of dance invention towards the end; but all dancers survived the test, although Margot Fonteyn's unabated freshness and sparkle were, perhaps, outstanding. Nothing could more emphasise her supremacy as a ballerina.

Because of its lack of emotional interest I do not believe this is the greatest of Ashton's works or one which will prove to have most staying power. But at his best Ashton's strength is not only in his dance invention, and he takes his place above all other English choreographers who compose in terms of pure dance just because he knows when to intensify the beauty and expressiveness of that dance by the contrast of dramatic gesture or actual immobility. The static figures of the Spectator in *Nocturne* and, at certain moments, of the Wanderer are the key to Ashton's greatness as a dance creator.

CHAPTER XIII

ROBERT HELPMANN AS CHOREOGRAPHER

THE maturity of mind which Robert Helpmann has been able to bring to his earliest ballets, partly owing to his late start as a choreographer and partly owing to his natural mental equipment born of wide tastes and theatrical knowledge, has already been mentioned earlier in this book, and the depth and versatility of his genius as a mime must be apparent from the foregoing record of some of his performances. He is an artist in that rare sense which Noverre recognised and panegyrised in David Garrick; one in whom a limitless range is allied with complete naturalness and eloquence of expression and an exceptionally convincing and varied command of make-up. "If there exist any man who cannot give a character to his face" wrote Noverre, with sublime disregard of the consequences, "he should leave the stage for ever"; an interdiction which would denude modern ballet of a good proportion of its most highly paid executants but which is at the root of Helpmann's pre-eminence as a dancer-artist.

In style and powers Helpmann probably more nearly approximates to Garrick, Noverre's ideal for the dancer-actor of the future, than any dancer since the publication of Noverre's book. Garrick, wrote Noverre, "always acted with his mind," and "to diction, delivery, fire, native wit and delicacy he united that rare gift for pantomimic expression which characterises the great actor and perfect comedian." A distinguished modern critic of acting, James Agate, has always tended to the view that, while Edmund Kean was indubitably the greatest English tragedian, Garrick's unique genius, though he was an artist of considerable tragic gifts unmatched in his own time, was as a comedian. To some extent this histrionic balance may be found eventually to apply to Helpmann; less in the ballet theatre, where through the medium of pure mime he has sometimes attained tragic expression of very great strength, than in drama. Here his sense of poetry and the *fey* helped him in the creation of a superb and darkly-

87

gleaming Oberon, a shimmering creature born of the night air, never mortal, which was unanimously acceded the greatest in living memory; but his Hamlet, a performance of immense cogency and pathos, suggested that his vocal bent will always be for the more sensitive and intellectual in tragedy, not for the heroic, though his power to suggest the macabre and almost Dostöevskian instinct for suffering and mental turmoil give an additional and perhaps stronger direction to his dramatic work.

In the legitimate theatre, however, although not in ballet, there are others of equal or greater tragic force, for at best Helpmann's limited experience makes it necessary at the moment to discuss his dramatic acting in terms of potentiality rather than achievement; but in character *range* and as a comedian he stands alone, his drollery and busy invention, particularly in the creation of old men, being of that now rare type in which the Grimaldi clown and character comedian meet in a riot of mingled folly, caricature and acute human observation.

Helpmann's work as dancer and actor is of the utmost relevance in any study of his choreography, for not only his dramatic instinct but also his intense feeling for "style" and "line" in classical dancing have had an important influence in shaping his ballet creations. For although in two of his greatest works, *Hamlet* and *Miracle in the Gorbals*, he has not used dancing on the points or the more obvious conventions of classic technique, both the individual dance movements and the group compositions have a strong feeling for classical "line" and the architecture of good painting. Helpmann has, indeed, a painter's eye in balancing his groups and a dramatist's sense of climax, and the importance of his dramatic background and wide musical and artistic interests in his formation as dancer and choreographer cannot be overestimated. Such broadening of outlook and intelligence is essential in the forming of the really great artist in ballet and will always be perceptible in the artist's work.

Helpmann's choreographic contribution to ballet, however, is something of far deeper moment than a mere re-introduction of the dramatic emphasis urged by Noverre and first brought into English ballet by Ninette de Valois. In his best works he has deliberately attempted a merging of mime and dance in a more fluid degree than ever before, with a complete negation of virtuoso dancing which he feels might break the continuity and style of the dramatic structure. In this he has many points of contact with Kurt Jooss, although his feeling for classic "line" and richer sense of the vertical in choreographic architecture give his compositions a more clear-cut complexity than Jooss's intentionally curved, supple, but less varied and geometrically patterned construction.

Expressiveness and beauty, not only in the individual movement but in relation to the whole design and action, are the key to Helpmann's ballets. Steps as such do not interest him, but the expression of a theme and details of psychology through movement, however simple, are for him an absolute necessity of choreographic creation. Helpmann's simplicity is never meaningless; he packs his ballets with meaning, sometimes extremely subtle meaning that escapes the eye of the unpractised onlooker, and welds the detail into a sustained sweep of dramatic narration. Above all he has that original twist of brain that in the best artists of all kinds, the ones nearest to genius, will give a theme an entirely personal and imaginative form. Neither as an artist nor as a man is Helpmann ordinary or predictable. He is variable in mood, impressionable, witty, quick in response, but with a hard core of commonsense that saves his work from any hint of pretentiousness and gives it a consistent, finely-planned unity of form. In no sense a copyist, either as interpreter or creator, he has had the intelligence to grasp and develop his own particular style and vision and at the same time, a rare quality in the original artist, to appreciate that his own is not the only possible creative style but merely a legitimate part of the rich and varied design that ballet must be if it is to remain a living and comprehensive art which appeals to many types of people and not just to a specialised and mentally restrictive *coterie*.

COMUS

WITH his passion for the traditions of the theatre and English poetic drama it was inevitable that Helpmann would turn to dramatic sources for the themes of his early ballets. *Comus* was not, strictly speaking, his first ballet, since in 1939 he had created for one performance of the Royal Academy of Dancing Production Club, to the music of Ravel's *La Valse*, a dance study for *corps de ballet* and two leading dancers which Wendy Toye completed when another engagement prevented his filling in the final details; but *Comus*, produced at the New Theatre on 14th January 1942, was his first creation for a permanent company and as such a work of remarkable maturity and completeness as well as expressive charm. Based on Milton's masque, first presented at Ludlow Castle in 1634 before the President of Wales, Lord Bridgewater, and charmingly designed to commemorate

an incident in which the two sons and young daughter of the Earl
(who played the parts of the Lady and her brothers in the performance)
had been benighted and lost in Haywood Forest, Herefordshire, it
brought into ballet the new element of lyric verse spoken for its own
fire and beauty and not as a descriptive accompaniment to the action.
A ballet is a bad ballet if speech is used to illustrate action the
choreographer has failed to make clear by movement, but Helpmann's
introduction of two of Milton's speeches in *Comus* had a different
purpose; it was a legitimate attempt to bring into ballet the spirit of
the English Masque, in which poetry, as well as music and dance, was
an essential element, and from which ballet in this country mainly
evolved. A temporary omission of the verse while Helpmann was
preparing to act in *Hamlet* the play did not seriously break the cohesion
of the ballet,but it did emphasise how effective the verse had been both
in dramatically pointing a static group and in helping to retain something of the lyrical beauty of Milton's original. Since the verse has
once again taken its place in the construction of the ballet Helpmann
has given the first speech, the invocation to night, a new emphasis by
keeping the movement of the surrounding Rout in a continuous flux.
The poetry of the language soars like a phœnix, limpid and seductive,
above the grotesque, erotic and constantly shifting group, and
Comus, like Jonson's Volpone, corrupts by the very loveliness of the
sheen he puts on evil. Both speeches are spoken by Helpmann with
authentic fire and music and his superb insolence, like an evil flame,
holds the stage. He is helped by a striking and beautiful costume,
the designer having conceived the son of Circe and Bacchus as a
Jacobean aristocrat, elegant to the fingertips and with a cluster of
vine leaves in his hair which would delight the heart of Hedda Gabler.
    That Helpmann was approaching choreography with a fresh and
unfettered outlook was apparent from the first moments of the ballet.
The dance of the Attendant Spirit has the effect of an animated statue,
the sculptural poses held and then merging one into the other. Based
on the classical technique, it demands unusual poise and balance in the
dancer and a *fey* authority which Margaret Dale beautifully gave it.
Throughout the ballet one is conscious of the graphic movement of
the arms which in Helpmann's choreography is as important always
as that of the feet. The Attendant Spirit leading the brothers to their
lost sister, the movements of searching, innocence and fear in the
dance of the Lady, the parallel lunge of swords, arms and feet in the
pas de deux of the Brothers, the variations of a swimming stroke in

the dances of Sabrina the river nymph—these are not only lovely in themselves, they illustrate both action and character. The entrance of Sabrina and her nymphs, their curving, wave-like movements suggesting the river's flow, is a moment of translucent beauty as lyrical as the verse and song from which it derives, and the Attendant Spirit draws them from their haunt with hands of quivering, bird-like magic.

In his handling of the Rout Helpmann showed less control, but a subsequent revision, with Comus borne on to the stage shoulder-high by his bacchanalian crew, has sharpened the effect of his first appearance and given the Rout the massed intricacy of pattern it lacked before. The pyramidal grouping of the final tableau has a painter-like construction, the entrances and exits of the characters are contrived with dramatic effortlessness, and in the second scene *pas de deux* between Comus and the Lady Helpmann shows a fine sense of contrast between figures in motion and a static grouped background. The eye is held continuously by the relevant characters and action, and Oliver Messel's exquisitely-coloured Van Dyck designs and Purcell's porcelain music give the ballet unusual artistic coherence.

John Hart and David Paltenghi gave to the virile choreography of the Brothers a dashing cavalier romanticism, teamwork and strength that unfortunately disintegrated after Hart was called into the Forces, and Moyra Fraser's attenuated height and long, beautiful hands have never been so effectively used as in the dances of Sabrina, although at first sight the part might seem to need a dancer of a less brittle and more flowing style. The loveliest performance of the Lady remains that of Margot Fonteyn, a study in innocence born not of ignorance but of spiritual integrity, fragile in grace, but with an inner strength evil cannot touch.

HAMLET

WITH *Comus* Helpmann established himself as a choreographer of grace and dramatic expressiveness; with *Hamlet*, produced four months later on 19th May 1942, he suddenly revealed the full tumult of his imagination in a work which, like the work of every truly original creative artist, was stamped with the imprint of the creator's own individual genius and demanded new standards of criticism by which it must be judged. The result was a critical controversy, involving the entire scope and direction of ballet as an art, which has still not entirely subsided, although the ballet has long since won a permanent place in the repertoire and by its own success and force of vision become accepted by many who were at first bewildered by its new and strongly mimic approach.

"Diversity of opinion about a work of art," wrote Wilde, "shows that the work is new, complex and vital," and *Hamlet*, like *Job* before it, has had to establish its right of existence against the inevitable reaction of the commonplace mind when confronted with anything outside its neatly-docketed code of rules: "This is not a ballet (or play, or novel, or piece of music)." Such criticism, of course, is founded on a quibble. By the three-Act formula Shakespeare's *Hamlet* is not a play, and by Clement Scott's conception of playwrighting Ibsen's *Ghosts* was not a social drama but a number of unpleasant things, not unconnected with the sewerage system, which would only occur to the chaste Toryism of the Victorian mind. Modern dramatic criticism has learned more flexibility of judgment, and the intelligent playgoer does not find it necessary to protest, because his own preference is for Shakespeare, that Ibsen and Tchehov are without merit as dramatists and their plays should not be performed. If it is to survive ballet, like the drama, must be conceived in terms of more than one style and form of construction. "Choreography" is far more than an arrangement of dance steps, and the choreographer must be judged by his composition as a whole, which includes mime, general pattern, grouping and musical understanding as well as dramatic narration or the expression of an idea. Mime is a perfectly legitimate element in ballet. It figures in classical works as well as in modern dramatic ballets, where it becomes a less stylised and more integral part of the dance and movement. Subjects such as *Job* and *Hamlet* cannot be conceived (unless the choreographer is totally lacking in a sense of style and artistic taste) in terms of technical virtuosity, but if dramatic themes are to be excluded from ballet on this account the art will become dangerously limited in scope. At a time when so many formless and repetitive ballets are being created it is essential that as vital and original a work as *Hamlet* is given its due, and the choreographer of mind and imagination full freedom of expression.

Hamlet is a ballet, and a fine one: mime and dance so smoothly blended that one is hardly conscious where one ends and the other begins, and both perfectly matching the theme and music. The emotional content of the music, Tchaikovsky's overture-fantasia composed for a production of the play in 1885, Helpmann has vividly expressed throughout, synchronising the dramatic and musical climaxes with an exciting sense of timing. Some of the choreography has unusual imagination: Ophelia's madness, her linked fingers and restless movement of arms and shoulders poignantly expressing her wandering mind and the plaintive phrases of the woodwind; Hamlet's accelerated crawl forward to the footlights, his face taut with horror at the Ghost's revelation, his hands pounding the floor; the tender and beautifully devised *pas de deux* with Ophelia; the passing and re-passing images of the Queen and Ophelia, the two merged in Hamlet's fevered consciousness; Hamlet's series of arrested turns *posés*, hands blindly to forehead, the pose magnificently accentuating the drum-beat.

Helpmann has welded his *corps de ballet* into patterns of moving diagonal lines which cleverly sustain the flow of action. He also gives them character: their sweeping bowing suggests the treacherous servility that dogged Hamlet in his uncle's Court. Their parallel lines excitingly build up the entrances and exits of the principal characters and they also underline the emotion, anticipate or echo the action, with the vivid unreality of a dream. There is an instance early in the ballet when linked revolving couples gradually fade from the stage, followed by Ophelia and the Queen interlaced in the same remote and circling motion. The effect is of a reflection repeated indefinitely in a mirror, a figurative translation of an idea Orson Welles treated literally at one moment in the film *Citizen Kane*.

This sense of the disturbed outline of a dream is imaginatively sustained throughout: Hamlet seems, at times, outside the action, an invisible spectator. The King and Queen make love over and around him, in the Play Scene; Ophelia's bier, on which the dead Queen terrifyingly lies, is swept out by the bearers over his very head. Helpmann's choice of theme, an expressionistic variation on Hamlet's:

"For in that sleep of death what dreams may come
When we have shuffled off this mortal coil
Must give us pause"

puts the ballet outside the range of formal Shakespearean criticism; yet it does, psychologically, illumine the play, as Kean acted, "by flashes of lightning." One might protest the emphasis is over-macabre, the omission of Horatio obscures the "sweet Prince"; but Hamlet's was a lonely mind, and in this friendless Prince the loneliness is terribly emphasised. The *pas de deux* with Ophelia, too, delicately suggests Hamlet's frustrated tenderness, that deep, unexpressed need for maternal affection which he misses in his mother. The confusion of these two characters in Hamlet's vision-haunted and dying brain brings out with a painful sharpness the way in which his feeling for Ophelia is poisoned by his disillusion with the Queen.

There is little justification, that I can see, in Shakespeare's text for the suggestion of an Œdipus complex (the Elizabethans had not read their Freud and the raging topic of intellectual conversation was the very different psychological problem raised by the *Treatise of Melancholie*), but balletically Helpmann has suggested it with sensitive insight. This nightmate emphasis on the subconscious suggests infinite choreographic possibilities; it is, in fact, the most interesting and revealing aspect of the ballet. The telescoping of Yorick and the Gravedigger into one figure further heightens the dream atmosphere and is brilliantly used to point Hamlet's morbid obsession with mortality; his rolling of the skull, and macabre return at Hamlet's death, are horrific touches. Other details make a curious impact on the mind: Hamlet sensing the Ghost's presence and being drawn backwards to him with an agonised and reluctant fascination; the Ghost pouring his tale into Hamlet's ear as Claudius poured the poison into his own; Hamlet's comparison of the hands of Ophelia and the Queen, inextricably blurred in his brain. But Helpmann's inexhaustible subtlety can only be fully appreciated after several visits to the ballet. The compression of *Hamlet* is as remarkable as its concentrated and impetuous drama, and every movement in it is significant. The false touches—there are very few—are false only to the Shakespearean purist and never to the atmosphere of the ballet as conceived.

Hamlet is a ballet that makes considerable mimic demands on the interpreters, including that power of moving and walking to music that surprisingly few dancers possess. The ill-omened beauty of Celia Franca's Queen, David Paltenghi's forceful and treacherous King, the Gravedigger of Leo Kersley and later Ray Powell, Margaret Dale's small Page sickened and frightened like a child at the sight of blood, all showed the increasing ability of the dancers in this company to build up a character, and the tragic helplessness and lurking terror that Margot Fonteyn gives to the part of Ophelia are completely in the spirit of the ballet. I have seen no stage actress express so sensitively the pitiful impotency of the character, too easily afraid, loving but helpless to understand Hamlet's suffering and need. In one gesture, a timid caress not quite daring to touch Hamlet's hair, she expresses Ophelia's whole tragedy. Laertes, a difficult because not strongly defined or explained character, is the part that most easily becomes a cypher, although the virility of John Hart, its creator, and the expressiveness of John Field later made it seem a definite part of the scheme of action.

Helpmann himself mimes the part of Hamlet with Renaissance intensity and that power of projecting atmosphere which only the great artist possesses. There is an unforgettable moment in this performance—the expression on his face when the Queen kisses him before the duel. Its sense of fleeting peace, of rest from turmoil, is strangely moving: one glimpses the true Hamlet in his terrible isolation and need for affection. Helpmann's performance has imagination, suffering and a striking mobility of face and hands; but a mere exploitation of the particular talents of an individual dancer the ballet certainly is not. It is a complete entity in which music, dramatic action, dancing and *décor* all cohere. Leslie Hurry's *décor* is the most exciting seen in ballet since Bakst's giddy perspective in *Scheherazade* and Helpmann's flair for stage production, notable in all his ballets, has aided him in the planning of lighting that eerily reflects the shifting phantasmagoria of the theme. A few performances without Helpmann confirmed the ballet to be a finely planned work which could still make an effect, even when weakly cast, by means of its beauty of line and perspective and dramatic velocity; but just as *Comus* suffered in style without his tortuous and lissom elegance, the dramatic balance of *Hamlet* is dependent, in the absence of any artist in ballet of comparable gifts, on his rare sensitivity and variety of expression. The measure of Helpmann's achievement in the part of Hamlet is his ability to preserve, even in this macabre distorted vision, a flash of lingering frustrated sweetness that links the character with the Shakespearean original.

THE BIRDS

HELPMANN'S following ballet, *The Birds*, produced also in 1942, proved the lightest and most insubstantial of his works, a *Wind in the Willows* of the ballet world and a happy little comedy for the younger dancers of the company, though in no sense a continuation or development of the dance-style he had used with such individuality and importance in *Hamlet*. The dancing was all purely classical and a refutation of the theory, much expressed after *Hamlet*, that Helpmann could only build a ballet around his own personality or in terms of dramatic mime. Simply, and without fuss, it translated bird movement into dance, from the grotesque pawing of the Hen, with a genuinely funny burlesque of the classical *developpé*, to the pert Cockney hop, run and *entrechats* of the Sparrows and the softer grace of the Doves;

and although the dance of the Dove and four attendant doves was weak and ragged, both musically and pictorially, it contained a charming bird pose, with foot tucked up and drooping head, that acted as a dove *motif* throughout the ballet. The romantic *pas de deux* of the Nightingale and the Dove was difficult technically but caught the mood of scene and music, and three of its inventions linger in the memory even now: a series of turns for the two dancers with a parallel diagonal sweep of the arms; a moment, poetically expressing the murmuring undercurrent of the music, when the Dove circled slowly round the Nightingale in grave, kneeling poses with bowed head; a final charming picture of the two nestling together beneath folded wings. Even the tragedy of the bird world was fleetingly touched on when the lovers, surprised by the Cuckoo, darted apart with quick alarmed movements of the head, and the Dove became instantly protective.

These little timid head movements formed an expressive part of the dancing of the Nightingale, and her motion of hands cupped to lips, as well as the brilliance of her spins, suggested the joyousness of song. Beryl Grey gave to this, her first created part, a shimmering iridescence and sweetness; but it was a virtuoso part requiring extremely careful partnering and there is no doubt Helpmann over-tried his dancers. Alexis Rassine, although a dancer of natural grace and beautiful arabesque "line," was not strong enough as partner or mime to give the *pas de deux* the assurance and suggestion of newly-awakened love it demanded, and Helpmann's later attempts to simplify the dance took away from its original spontaneity and "line." The Sparrows of Margaret Dale and Joan Sheldon had a choirboy innocence in mischief that was cheekily disarming, and Moyra Fraser, an over-tall dancer who had not always been too happily cast, scored a distinct success as the Hen, playing with a first-rate sense of comedy and timing. Palma Nye later played the part with strong comic invention but lacked the same chicken-like delicacy of neck-stretching and tread. It was in the creation of this character, and the deliberate burlesque for Cuckoo and Hen of the earlier *pas de deux* of the Nightingale and the Dove, that Helpmann imprinted his own personality on the ballet. The fun was entirely his own, and the exquisite Chinese fairy-tale *décor* of Chiang Yee and Respighi's attractive selection of bird music fitted the ballet like a glove. *The Birds* made a useful small addition to the comedy side of the repertoire (*Façade* had long been slightly frayed from overwork) and some of us were sorry when it faded out of the repertoire, leaving only the glint of a golden feather, like the Firebird in Fokine's ballet, behind.

MIRACLE IN THE GORBALS

CREATIVE art is the outward expression of the inner vision of the artist, and the impression of life created by the artist through his work will vary according to the originality and intensity of that vision. Turner, Cézanne and Van Gogh, painting an identical landscape, would produce pictures as totally different in effect as the ballet of *Hamlet* by Nijinska must have been from the ballet of *Hamlet* by Robert Helpmann. The success of the artist's work depends not on the "truth" of his vision—truth in art is many-sided—but on his power of projecting that vision into the minds of others. Helpmann, by an imaginative use of a highly individual but consistent choreographic style, achieved this magnificently in the case of *Hamlet* and in *Miracle in the Gorbals*, produced at the Princes Theatre on 26th October 1944, he reverted to the form of expression, the dramatic fusion of mime and dance, which he established in *Hamlet* but deserted in *The Birds*. The result is a work of vital and moving power and one of the most significant ballets produced in our time.

The Ballets Jooss have shown that contemporary subjects may be expressed through the medium of the dance, though always in their case with a strain of satire or stylisation. *Miracle in the Gorbals*, as savage in its criticism of life as *The Green Table* or Synge's *Playboy of the Western World*, is purely realistic in conception and proves that a modern theme may be realised by a classical company with equal dramatic force and a still richer sense of character and choreographic counterpoint. In spite of its realistic approach the ballet is, in effect, a modern morality: its theme the simple one of a second coming of the Christ to a Glasgow slum, his raising of a girl suicide from the dead, his conversion of a prostitute, rejection, and violent death at the instigation of a modern Caiaphas.

The ballet has been criticised as melodrama, but this criticism can only be accepted if it is recognised that melodrama may form an element in the greatest works of the theatre: *Hamlet*, *King Lear* and *Macbeth* as well as *The Rake's Progress* and *Petrouchka*. What raises melodrama to the plane of art is the quality of the material used by the artist: poetry in the case of the Elizabethan playwright, choreography in the case of the modern ballet creator. Helpmann has handled his theme with reverence, poignancy and a teeming detail of character and incident recalling Ninette de Valois more than any other choreo-grapher. His brawling slum-street atmosphere of toughs, street girls, swarming urchins and pub-crawlers, with its dynamic elements of Irish and Scotch, is finely established, and although at first it seems that the ballet may prove more brilliant "stage production" than dance and the over-crowding tenements of Edward Burra's setting may cramp Helpmann in his groupings, the doubt is quickly dispelled. From the entrance of the Suicide, in an *adagio* expressive in its despair and requiring great bodily flexibility and balance, Helpmann takes a firm grasp of his crowd and only once again, in the rushing to and fro at the news of the girl's death, tends to lose it.

In *Hamlet* the dream atmosphere was conveyed by deliberately formal patterns and a *corps de ballet* which danced in unison, as a single and inhuman entity. In *Miracle in the Gorbals* the dance orchestration is altogether richer, the pyramid groupings are strikingly plastic and there is increased mastery of lifts and pliant movement. Details of scene and character stand out vividly in retrospect: the Suicide's mute gesture of appeal to the heedless and drunken women of the crowd, and her recoil in revulsion, the one key to her tragedy, from a man who grasps her by the arm; the jaunty, self-satisfied gait of a tough coming from the room of the Prostitute; the eloquent figure of a girl leaning frightened against the wall as the mob shuffle back, with bowed heads, and part suddenly to reveal the limp figure of the drowned girl; the momentary awed stillness as the Christ, with a gesture of austere beauty, raises the Suicide from the dead; her delicate little Scotch reel of grave delight as the life returns to her limbs, and the primitive worship of the mob lashed to an intensifying rhythm of negro spiritual ecstasy and jitterbug frenzy, a reaction instinctive to such people in such a district; a child's excited and unmoved miming of the girl's drowning; the flash of pain on Helpmann's face, almost the only expression he allows himself in a performance of stylised restraint, when an urchin spits at him; the arm poised to strike and slash of the razor that ends the suffering of this new Christ; the dead arms outstretched, stark and pitiable, as the Beggar, a sudden figure of compassion, holds the shattered body in his arms; the covering of the torn face with the scarf which had covered the face of the drowned girl before the miracle; the final moving simplicity of the departure of the two women, the converted harlot and the suicide, with one lingering backward glance at the motionless body on the ground. The scene of the murder has a Renaissance and almost unbearable violence, a savage comment on an age which has produced its torturers and hired thugs in direct descent from the world of Machiavelli's *The Prince*. The agony of this Crucifixion is unsentimentalised, the mob, shallow in its emotions, has the capriciousness and brutality of Synge's peasants. It is against this pitilessness and social squalor that Helpmann and the author of the ballet, Michael Benthall, are crying out; the religious illustration is used to drive home their pity and horror. It is not a complete picture, the generosity and hospitality, even the deeper misery, of the poor are not touched on; these are subjects for some future choreographer and scenarist, and a ballet less bitter than this. The important point is that ballet has proved itself as vital a medium as the drama or the novel for the depiction of modern life, and produced a work which, for all its brutal force, has genuine beauty and compassion.

Helpmann has been admirably served by his dancers and the Sadler's Wells Company as a team show here the power of creating low-life character that informs their work in *The Rake's Progress*. Celia Franca's beauty in the character of the Magdalen burned with a sensual and later spiritual flame, and her sickened contempt of the Official was subtly mimed. David Paltenghi as this repressed and bitter Caiaphas gave his finest performance to date and in his study of his hands after the murder graphically conveyed the man's realisation of his own sin. Pauline Clayden as the Suicide had grace and genuine grief, Leslie Edwards gave a performance of perfect artistry as the Beggar, a beautifully conceived character combining something of the Russian "innocent" and the Irish fiddler, and Julia Farron's gum-chewing street girl and Moyra Fraser's bleary "char" were sharply touched in. Gordon Hamilton's Dead End Kid had the young-old look of the undernourished and disturbingly suggested the blight of arrested mental development in the slum; it needed only a trace more viciousness for us to believe that it is from this material that the adult tough and razor-slasher is bred. Moira Shearer and Alexis Rassine brought a lyrical grace-note into the cacophony of the slum and Jean Bedells as the girl's mother, shrilly depicted in the music, had a blousy aggressiveness. Edward Burra's setting and costumes capture the colour and squalor of the district and his drop curtain, a russet ship rearing from the docks against a clouded iron-grey sky, is in his boldest style. Arthur Bliss's music is rhythmical and atmospheric, a beautiful and exciting score with a dramatic accentuation of the drum beat, and Helpmann has matched it with his usual sensitive correlation of ear and vision. Helpmann's own performance of the Christ, a slight and youthful figure in worker's clothes and sandals, has a passionless beauty and the El Greco quality of the face gives the character exactly the right sense of having stepped from another world and period.

Miracle in the Gorbals brings ballet completely away from the fairy tale into the heart of the life, character and problems of our time. By any standards it is a landmark in ballet. The courage of the Sadler's Wells Company in producing it shows the vigorous and progressive outlook of the English National Ballet, and its enthusiastic reception by audiences is an encouraging indication that the public mind is alive to new dramatic and social ideas in ballet and not bound to escapism and prettiness.

ADAM ZERO

TO Robert Helpmann fell the distinction of being the first English choreographer of our time to create a ballet at Covent Garden, and no new work could have more significantly matched the occasion than his *Adam Zero*, produced at the Opera House on 10th April 1946. For this ballet not only carries one stage further the progress of English ballet along new lines of choreographic thought and creation, it also makes bold and imaginative use of all the mechanical resources of that great and lavishly equipped stage.

Adam Zero is an allegory, told, as the modern American play *The Skin of Our Teeth* was told, in terms of a theatrical performance in which the illusional devices of the stage are stripped bare to the eyes of the audience, and the play or ballet is built up before us in an atmosphere which is an exciting blend of rehearsal, creative composition and artistic completion. The method is not new in the theatre —in its simplest form it exists in the centuries-old theatre of China— but Helpmann's adaptation of it to ballet is free and original, and his parallel of the cycle of man's life from birth to death with the creation of a new ballet in the theatre is achieved with an emotional cogency and pliability of design that are equally remarkable.

It is impossible to capture in words the spellbinding poignancy of this symbol of contemporary man, born, as a ballet and dancer are born, in the stress and toil of an empty theatre; dancing through the lyric and primitive spring of life to the triumphant classic splendour of summer's heat; touched by the first chill of autumn and the fateful application of the make-up box that heralds old age; superseded by

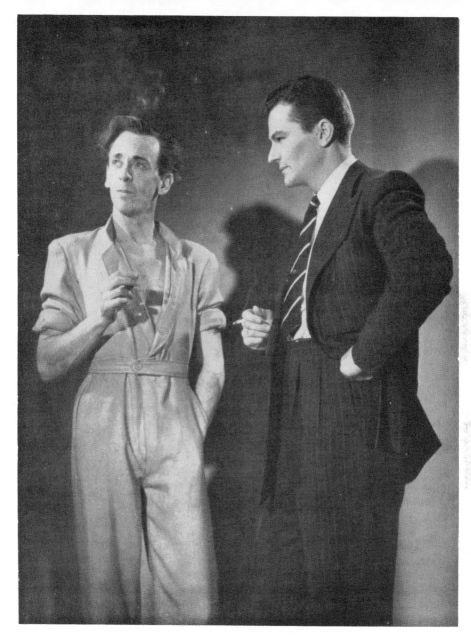

Choreographer and Scenarist
Robert Helpmann and Michael Benthall.

Plate XXIX

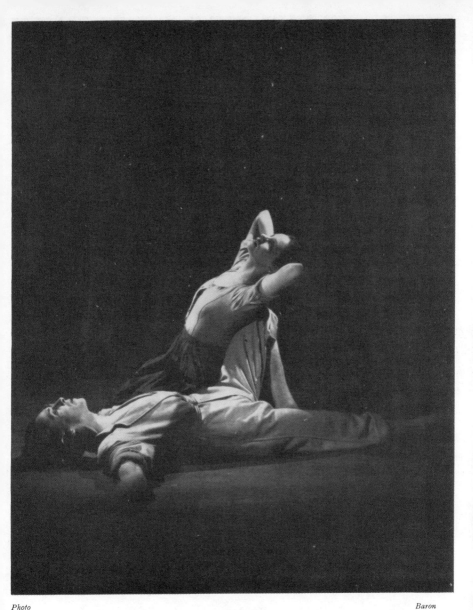

Adam Zero
Adam and his First Love: Robert Helpmann and June Brae

Plate XXX

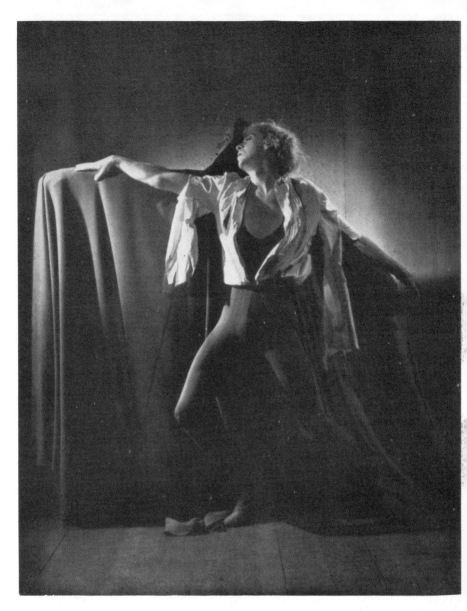

Photo

Baron

Adam Zero
Adam and Death: Robert Helpmann and June Brae

Plate XXXI

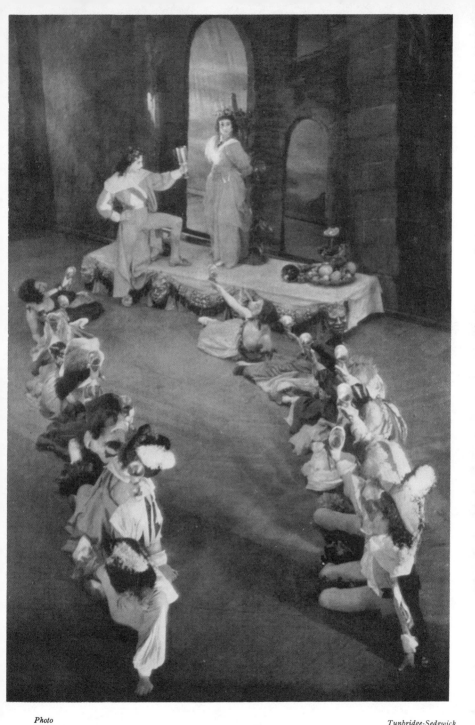

Comus
Drama and "line" in grouping: Scene with Helpmann and Fonteyn

Plate XXXII

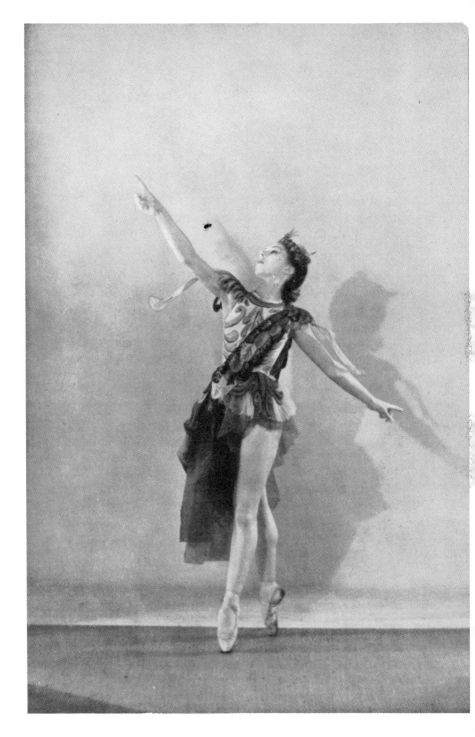

Photo

Anthony

Comus
Margaret Dale as the Attendant Spirit

Plate XXXIII

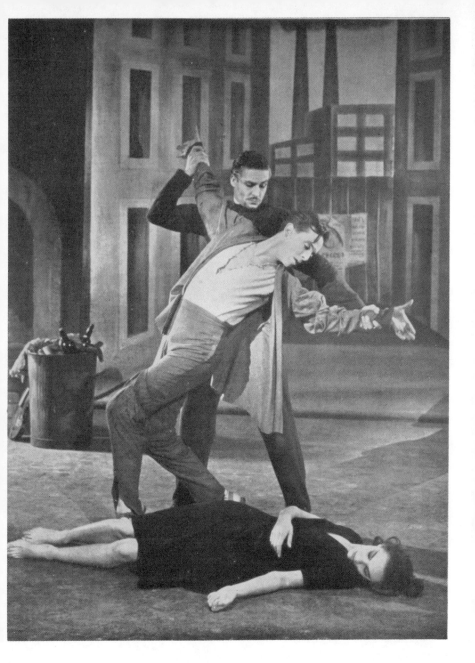

Photo
Edward Mandinian

Miracle in the Gorbals
Raising of the Suicide: David Paltenghi, Robert Helpmann
and Pauline Clayden

Plate XXXIV

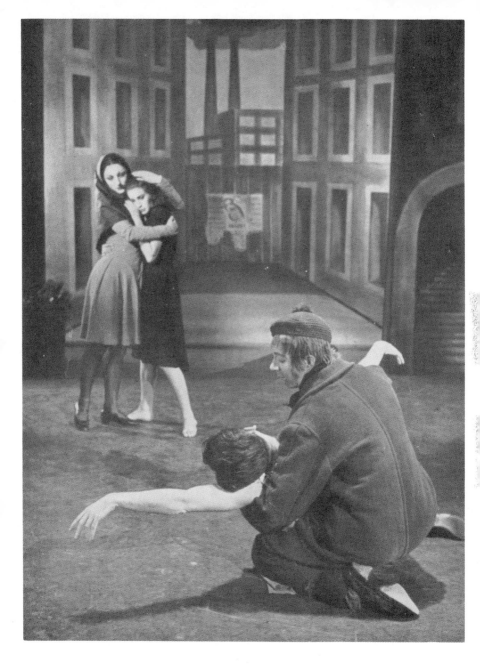

Photo

Edward Mandinian

Miracle in the Gorbals
Death of the Stranger: Celia Franca, Pauline Clayden,
Robert Helpmann and Leslie Edwards.

Plate XXXV

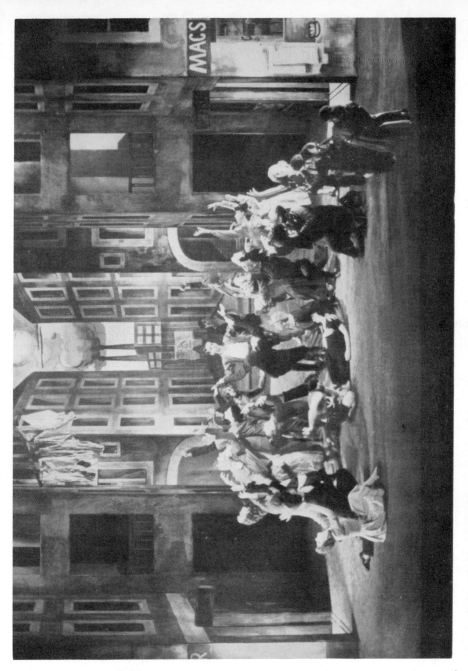

Miracle in the Gorbals.
Group in revival scene. *Décor* by Edward Burra.

Plate XXXVI

the younger generation who is both son and understudy; caught up in the mad degeneracy of the jazz-age that mocked and danced as the world flared into destruction; finally crawling through the bleak winter of our Belsens to the protective arms of Death.

It is marked by subtle touches that reinforce yet, by some magic, never overcrowd the theme, from the cut skein of life of the man's three Fates (Designer, Wardrobe Mistress and Dresser), and the sleeping Church to whom he turns unavailingly for solace, to the appearance of his son and daughter (a bitter comment on the brotherhood of man) as guards in the scene in Belsen. Nothing in Helpmann's own performance is more moving than the eager, unrealising joy with which, as the young Adam, he takes from the Fates the first discarded strand of his life, or in old age his slow shuffle on his knees to the Priest and feeble attempt to rub out with one shaking finger the last chalked zero on the blackboard of his life. Man in this ballet is the victim of his Fates: he has no final responsibility for his own destiny. He is a symbol of the individual, achieving a little, losing it, enjoying and suffering blindly, crushed by the inexorable march of time from which there is no escape and by the dark history of man's persecution of man.

"As flies to wanton boys are we to the gods,
They kill us for their sport."

If the figure loses in nobility it gains in pathos; and what critic of to-day dare say, with the bones in the gas chambers of devastated Europe before him, that there is no tragic drama without personal responsibility?

The ballet has a magnificent inevitability of plan and design for which the scenarist, Michael Benthall, must be held responsible; even the "election" parody, which seems irrelevant, falls into place when the rags of the starved in Belsen repeat the symbol "Vote for Adam Zero," and the bitter harvest of modern politics is laid bare. And the theme of the nothingness of man's individual life is rounded off with a less unhopeful sense of the continuity of life as a whole; the wheel comes full circle, and on the empty stage with its watchful dancers we witness a recapitulation and a new birth.

The ballet is brought to life by a striking correlation of design, music, stage production and dance forms. The lighting, beautiful throughout, throws into relief both Helpmann's choreography and Roger Furse's designs, most notably in the jazz scene, which with its intoxicating rhythms and leaping flames has a quality almost dæmonic, and the scene of "Spring" where the colours are exquisitely blended. The cyclorama, dwarfing the dancers beneath it, is nowhere more impressive than when it stretches, an endless wintry wasteland of shifting cloud, behind the scarlet-cloaked figure of Death, and Helpmann's dance arrangement fully exploits the pity and the majesty, as well as the visual beauty, of this scene in which Death enfolds the dying man in arms like wings of enveloping flame.

Using every dance convention, primitive, acrobatic, modern and classic, Helpmann has achieved a choreographic pattern that coincides with the heights and depths of civilised life. The difficult scenes of the birth and concentration camp are arranged with eloquent restraint, the birth scene attaining, with the support of Arthur Bliss's triumphant and poignant music, an extraordinary sense of the miracle of life through the mother's pain. The revelation of the naked man-child, Adam, in the compact position of a baby at birth, is strangely impressive, and the abounding energy and grace of his youth revealed in choreography that includes virile "lifts" and a sensational leap from the rostrum on to the outstretched arms of the youths beneath. The "Marriage" scene that follows is perhaps the loveliest in the ballet; perfect in musicality and pattern, it has a spring-like tenderness and religious awe, and a use of "lift" and embrace that transposes erotic feeling on to a purely poetic plane. Lines of dancers meet and interlace with the man lifted prostrate over the girl, youths, moving slowly in a circle, cover him with a grave, wheeling motion of the arms, groups of kneeling girls and youths rise and fall to the music in a serene counterpoint. And while the girl lifts her face in ecstasy to the sun, on the man's face as he looks at her there is a sudden uncomprehending sadness, a premonition. For as in ancient myths of the Earth-Mother, the same woman in this ballet is not only birth-giver and wife but also Death. Man comes from the earth, and returns to it.

Musically this is Helpmann's most complex and brilliant ballet; his use of dancers at barre and practice in the opening scene shows a varied rhythmic undulation and "line" that can only be compared to orchestral harmony, and in the classical scene, the highest artistic form of the dance matching the high summer of a man's life, contrapuntal timing gives a new effect to Petipa-like "dives" and pirouettes. Arthur Bliss's music, rich in colour and texture, gives dramatic beauty to the whole, and one's only criticism is that the jazz scene and Dance of Death are both a trifle over-long.

Helpmann as Adam progresses superbly from the golden vitality and charm of youth to the wasted martyrdom of age; if one would single out any one moment in his performance it is the expression on his face when the costume of the dancer is snatched from him, and the hard strokes of the Stage Director's chalk put the first grey in his hair. There is prevision here, and a helpless pathos as he moves slowly backstage with his cat in his arms: the line of his shoulders speaks. The charmingly-conceived part of the Cat, supply acrobatic and affectionate, was deliciously created by Pauline Clayden, and Gillian Lynne as the Daughter, Leslie Edwards as the Priest and David Paltenghi as the Stage Director (an unobtrusive but perfect performance that was invaluable to the ballet) were ideally cast.

Throughout the ballet woman is both Creator and Destroyer: Choreographer, Wife, Mistress and Death. June Brae, returning to the stage after several years' absence, played all parts with an artistry that ranged easily from the lyric to the seductive and awe-inspiring. Only in the classical scene did she fail, and this was in the circumstances understandable; but in poetry and intensity of feeling, and expressiveness of movement, the performance was sufficiently remarkable.

Adam Zero is a ballet only Robert Helpmann could have successfully handled. Original without pretentiousness, it is a great and astonishing work to have been produced in only four weeks of rehearsals by a man who was, at the time, still weak from a long illness, and like Helpmann's other works it has once again brought ballet to a new and wider public, which includes representatives of other arts and professions as well as people who had never before realised ballet's scope as a reflection of life. It is impossible to look on this infusion of new blood and intelligence into the ballet audience as anything but a good thing; it has opened up to the creator fresh possibilities of expression, and released ballet from the narrow limits of appeal imposed by the specialised *coterie* group. In this popularising of the art Helpmann's ballets have played an undeniable and valuable part.

With Ashton's *Dante Sonata* and *The Wanderer* Helpmann's *Hamlet*, *Miracle in the Gorbals* and *Adam Zero* represent the outstanding achievement of ballet in this country since 1939. It may or may not be significant that in three of these five works no use is made of pointwork, but certainly English ballet, while fully maintaining classical traditions through Ashton's other ballets and regular performance of the "classics," is developing a wide variety of styles and is no longer bound to express itself through conventional dance technique, though this forms the essential basic training of all its dancers and choreographers.

Helpmann's aim, expressed in an address to the Royal Academy of Dancing soon after the production of his ballet *Hamlet*, has been "to adjust the conventional mime of the Classical School and combine it with the movement, thereby evolving a type of mimetic-movement which should be more understandable to a modern audience." The echo of Fokine's self-confessed endeavour "to replace gestures of the hands by mimetic of the whole body" is interesting. All the constructive thinkers of ballet from Noverre onwards have felt something the same need and in Helpmann's creation both as dancer and choreographer thought takes as significant a part as instinct. If ballet is understood as an artistic whole of which the dance is an integral but not predominant part it is essential that it should do so.

CHAPTER XIV

SADLER'S WELLS AND THE CLASSICS

GISELLE

IT was with the production of *Giselle* on 1st January 1934, with Alicia Markova and Anton Dolin in the leading parts, that the Sadler's Wells Ballet thus early in its career established its policy of preserving in its repertoire, as an indispensable technical background for its dancers and choreographers, all the principal classical ballets which could be reconstructed in their entirety. *Giselle*, the sole survivor of French romanticism, was followed shortly afterwards by the Tchaikovsky-Petipa *Casse Noisette*, and on 20th November 1934 by the first production outside Russia of the original four-Act version of *Lac des Cygnes*, the finest Russian expression of romantic classicism which in its more usual second Act version had for some time been danced by Markova for the company. A two-Act version of *Coppélia* (with Lydia Lopokova and later Ninette de Valois as Swanhilda) was in the repertoire of the company from a still earlier period, although the little-known third Act, reconstructed by Nicholas Sergueff, was not added until 1940. The production on 2nd February 1939 of *The Sleeping Princess*, a triumph for Margot Fonteyn as the first productions of *Giselle* and *Lac des Cygnes* had been for Markova, gave the Wells a full repertoire of the three principal Russian and the only surviving French classics.

The value to the company in its earliest formative years of a Russian-trained ballerina of the status of Markova cannot be overestimated; without her neither *Giselle* nor *Lac des Cygnes* could have been added to the repertoire, and as the first English dancer to play the part of Giselle she made ballet history. Later she danced the part for a Russian company at Drury Lane and since the war, again with Dolin as partner, she has achieved the greatest triumph of her career in performances of the same ballet for the Ballet Theatre of America. Belonging to the Taglioni type of dancer, her imponderable lightness gave an almost transparent spirituality to the second Act and since the great dancer, in her most active dancing years, rarely fails to progress artistically it is possible that when Markova dances the part of Giselle again in England we shall find her performance enriched both emotionally and technically.

After Markova left the Sadler's Wells Company in 1935 the rôle of ballerina was gradually assumed by a very young dancer, Margot Fonteÿn, and it is through her rapidly maturing and deeply touching performance, supported with great artistry and selflessness by Robert Helpmann, that *Giselle* has in recent years reached what will probably prove to be its high-water level of popularity in England.[1] A dancer of exquisite qualities of "line," musicality and sensitive expression, she has built up in *Giselle* a characterisation of such insight and range of mood that her first Act is considered by some to be the best dramatically since that of Pavlova. Charming, gay, but dangerously highly-strung, her Giselle is not a normal village girl but one in whom a nervous impressionability, easily swayed by happiness or grief, and a single-minded devotion of unmistakable gentleness and depth, lead logically to mental breakdown when she believes her lover is lost to her. With her dark eyes, large and luminous with joy or fear, her pale mobile face, her slenderness and mercurial grace, she has already something of the *fey* immateriability of the Wili she is to become. There are many perceptive touches in this performance; her timid fingering of Bathilde's silk gown, wide-eyed with delight, her distracted searching of Loys's face for reassurance, her shy but passionate love for him which one feels even in the wraith of the second Act, with its protective pity and tender last gesture, her hand sliding down his cheek as he lowers her into the grave. Her Mad scene is moving because it shows a mind with glimmerings of lucidity, the same quality that makes her Ophelia touching, and her sudden recognition of her lover, with the full horror of comprehension, just before her death, has profound pathos.

Fonteyn's lack of elevation is felt by some to mar her dancing of the second Act, but it is always worth remembering that the part of Giselle was originally created, not by the aerial Taglioni, but by Carlotta Grisi, whose dancing according to Gautier had in this part "incomparable grace, lightness, intrepidity and vigour," who was "nature and artlessness personified," but whose *jetés* do not appear

[1] The reaction to classicism after the death of Diaghileff, whose production of *The Sleeping Princess* in 1921 was a costly failure, is a curious aspect of modern ballet history. When *Giselle* was in the programme in the early days at Sadler's Wells the audience, in the words of a wittier member of the company, "*fought to get out of the theatre!*" It is now the ballet for which, after *Lac des Cygnes* and *The Sleeping Beauty*, it is most difficult of all to obtain a seat.

to have been excessively commented on by contemporary critics. Through her delicate artistry and light, unhurried softness of movement, Fonteyn achieves a suggestion of remoteness that yet glows with a spiritualised sweetness and affection; her dancing shows fluent ease and control and her slow *pirouettes en attitude*, ending in a faultlessly poised arabesque, in her first Act variation are studies in balance, precision and style. The complete spontaneity of her dancing in the first Act gives freshness and sparkle to the whole scene; it is dancing for the love of it, without the slightest hint of classical exhibitionism. Her *spirit* dances, and infects her lover with its quick shining gaiety.

Helpmann's response here and throughout the ballet is of unobtrusive help to his partner and his Albrecht, always a little graver, older, sensible of her child-like trust and need for protection, is a characterisation of a sympathy and restraint unequalled in our time. Here, as in all the classical ballets, he has the instinctive elegance of the true aristocrat, with the result that when Giselle draws him into her dances one feels a charming vivacity that springs from a sense of release, a release from the formalities of a Court. This Albrecht's feeling for Giselle is genuine and sincere, and there is indeed little in the text to justify the identification of the character with that of an ordinary seducer. The engagement to Bathilde was probably forced on the young man by political convenience, and this Albrecht in his dignity and troubled reserve when she appears suggests respect but no love. Some sense, however, of his responsibility to Giselle he has, and the momentary concern in his face, and his instant reassurance, when Giselle collapses in tears after the plucking of the flower is a protective reaction in which one feels a disturbed consciousness of deception and anxiety for Giselle. Helpmann reacts to a situation on the stage with every fibre of body and brain; movement, gesture and facial expression are completely correlated and indivisible. Nowhere is this more apparent than in this ballet; in his quick start of recognition, query and alarm when Giselle shows him the necklace given her by Bathilde; his immobile realisation of death as her hand slips limply through his fingers; his suggestion of suppressed but unabated grief in the second scene, together with a feeling for poetry and atmosphere that enhances Giselle's intangibility, her phantom-like escape from his embrace.

Essentially a romantic-style classical dancer, Helpmann is at his best in this ballet, where his purity of "line," *ballon* and flowing grace of movement give the second act dancing a plastic beauty. His double turns in the air have a smoothness and perfection of finish unequalled in England to-day, and he is alone in his ability to make this scene's one virtuoso solo fit into the lyrical scheme of the dancing as a whole. The Russian-style flamboyance and strength that has sometimes been given by the *danseur noble* to this ballet is alien to its period and character. Helpmann's performance is probably nearer than that of most modern dancers to the original of Lucien Petipa, to whom, if contemporary lithographs are to be believed, he bears some physical resemblance. "Petipa was graceful, passionate and touching," wrote Gautier in his letter to Heine after the first performance of *Giselle*. "A mime of intelligence," he commented on the same dancer later, "he always fills the stage and does not neglect the slightest detail." Both descriptions might have been written of Helpmann.

The choreographic excellence of *Giselle* is not confined to the expressive and technically exacting dances arranged for the two principal characters. The *corps de ballet* dances, far more than in the case of the later Russian classical ballets, are threaded naturally into the action and in the second Act particularly take a necessary part in the drama. The graceful simplicity of pattern in the first-Act dances of the villagers is such that the use of classical pointwork does not destroy their artlessness and spontaneity, and the *ballottés* and *jetés* of Giselle and her lover bring to the scene a springing lightness of heart. The second Act *pas de deux* of Giselle and Albrecht are carefully designed to express her spirituality, and yet, in their swaying supported arabesques and elusive contacts, in the pity and seductiveness of Giselle's gesture to her exhausted lover, there is a suggestion of earthly sensuousness raised to a plane of abstract poetry. Danced with the complete mutual sympathy of a Fonteyn and a Helpmann the whole Act becomes a love duet of poignant evanescence. The frigid heartlessness expressed in the lines and poses of the Wilis dramatically overshadows the two dancers, and their influence in the action, particularly in the tearing apart of the two lovers who are yet drawn back to each other by an irresistible magnetism, could be more strongly marked in modern performances of the ballet, in which the second Act tends as far as the *corps de ballet* is concerned to become a lovely but emotionless study in pure dance. A few of the dramatic points of the original scenario, based by Gautier and Saint-Georges on some ideas of the poet Heine, might also be reintroduced into the ballet with some gain to the clarity of the plot. Apart from this the Sadler's Wells production of this ballet has always shown a sincere understanding of its spirit and period, without the fatal sophistication that has ruined the atmosphere in some modern performances.

The romantic style of the choreography seems more easily assimilated by English dancers than the glittering virtuosity of Petipa classicism, and the pattern and feeling of the dances have always been preserved. Among the performances of the Queen of the Wilis Pamela May's ice-cold cruelty and Celia Franca's gossamer elevation and musicality have been notable. Lacking the straightness of knee and strength of pointwork of the pure classical dancer, Franca is a born dancer of such natural grace, poetry and style that she succeeded here, and as a leading Swan in *Lac des Cygnes*, where many more strictly virtuoso dancers have failed. Her intelligence gives her, in addition, a dramatic range that has been brilliantly utilised by Helpmann and opened up to her some of the finest acting parts in the modern repertoire. The variations of the two leading Wilis, Zulme and Moyna, have also had a high standard of execution in Wells performances, and the charming *pas de quatre* for the young villagers in the first Act has been consistently well danced.

Giselle, as danced by Fonteyn and Helpmann, reaches the highest interpretative standard in Sadler's Wells productions of the classics. During 1944 the two principal parts were danced for the first time in seven years by other dancers of the company; a delicate experiment since *Giselle*, at one time reserved for the great dancer as the crown to her career, is a period piece that tends to show its mechanics of construction unless portrayed by artists of emotional maturity and depth. Beryl Grey's height was against her in the first scene, and she lacked the quicksilver contrast of gaiety and foreboding that leads naturally to the girl's madness; but the childlike simplicity of her Mad scene had its own pathos and she brought to her second Act dancing a quality, at once wistful and remote, that denotes the instinctive artist. Alexis Rassine as Albrecht showed unexpected progress as a mime and gave a performance of youthful impetuosity and charm. He danced the difficult second Act variations with crispness, spring and improved finish, and with a little more fluidity in the *enchaînements*, and providing he can keep his acting fresh and sincere, this will be a *danseur noble* performance of some quality. It must still be recognised, however, that *Giselle* is a ballet that by tradition belongs to the great and finished artist, to the Pavlovas and Spessivitsevas, and too frequent performance by lesser dancers, as is happening in England to-day, cannot fail to damage its fragile texture.

LE LAC DES CYGNES

THE production of *Lac des Cygnes* on 7th September 1943, with
new scenery and costumes by Leslie Hurry, was the most notable
event in the history of Sadler's Wells performances of this ballet since
the original full-length production with Markova in 1934 and Margot
Fonteyn's first appearance in the dual rôles of Odette-Odile. For long
this ballet had relied on the brilliance of the ballerina to lift it into
the plane of the spectacular to which the ballets of the Maryinsky
Theatre truly belong; now for the first time Sadler's Wells gave to a
production of a Russian classical ballet the magnificence which is
Petipa's heritage, together with an artistic taste which was probably
lacking, in an equal degree, in the original St. Petersburg production.
The use of artists who were something more than efficient theatre
designers was not customary in Petipa's own day, and in this production his ballet becomes for the first time a unified entity of music,
choreography and *décor* on the lines of collaboration developed
much later in the ballets presented by Diaghileff.

The Russian Ballet's first appearance in Europe created a *furore* at
least as much due to its scenic artists as to its dancers and choreographer, and after a period during which the artist's status suffered a
decline it seems to have fallen to the English Ballet to revive Diaghileff's policy of bringing outstanding contemporary artists into the
theatre. Robert Helpmann's discovery and employment of Leslie
Hurry for his ballet *Hamlet* may prove to be the most significant
happening in ballet on the artistic side since Bakst's *Scheherazade*
revolutionised the colour sense of the West. The richness of the colour
scheme in Hurry's scenery and costumes for *Lac des Cygnes* does in
fact make the comparison with Bakst fairly apt, but here, as in *Hamlet*,
this young artist has shown an individuality of style and imagination
that brings something quite new and exciting into ballet design.

Hurry's achievement in *Lac des Cygnes* has been to combine his
surréalism with the traditions of classical ballet and the Russian
fairy tale. His mask of burning brass for the magician Von Rothbart
captures the terror and splendour of Russian wizardry which Gont-
scharova achieved *en masse* in *L'Oiseau de Feu*, and his scenery throughout has remarkable co-ordination, so that the whole fantasy seems to
unfold itself in a land shadowed by magic. Deep glowing blues and
greens are the basis of this land's colour, and the swan *motif* haunts
lake, forest and palace like a lovely and sinister ghost. Hurry's second
Act *décor*, a moon-hazed maëlstrom dominated by the image of a swan,

is a new and imaginative conception of the swan lake and in his palace scene, a fine piece of perspective draughtsmanship combining the Gothic arch, the perpendicular column and a delicate fan tracery roof, the costumes suddenly brighten the magic-filled atmosphere with a flash of white and scarlet, the Russian colour for weddings. Odile, in gold-encrusted black, stands out as a baleful and glittering figure of evil and the only unsatisfactory costumes are those for the Spanish dance, which lack national emphasis.

The best tribute to this *décor* is that it is worthy of Tchaikovsky's music and the Ivanov-Petipa choreography, with its well-defined contrast of spectacular *adagio*, variations and *divertissement* in the third Act and romanticism of feeling in the second and fourth. In the great *pas de deux* of the second Act Ivanov broke new ground through his realisation that Tchaikovsky's music demanded a richer dance orchestration than was traditional in the classical *pas de deux* of the period, and instead of clearing the stage for the two principal dancers he has used the *corps de ballet* as a fluid counterpoint and interruption of their dance. The fourth Act, although short, has the same beauty of style and grouping, the arrangement of line in the final tableau having a lyric simplicity and the mime passages of the doomed lovers, if adequately performed, genuine pathos and suspense. Tchaikovsky's music, although less well-known than that for the second Act, is also here at its finest. The performances of the Sadler's Wells *corps de ballet* clearly reveal the mobile patterns of the choreography and the third Act *pas de trois*, a fine study in classic technique, was danced with excellent precision on the first night of this production by Alexis Rassine, Margaret Dale and Joan Sheldon. This *pas de trois* has had some good performances in the past (that of John Field, clean in line and *batterie*, was at the time of his call-up becoming notable) but it has been too often treated as a technical "try-out" for inexperienced dancers. In Russia and in the Diaghileff ballet it was not considered below the status of the finest classical technicians, including the ballerinas, of the company.

Among the minor performances Ray Powell's old German tutor was a genuine character, amusingly observed but never losing the sense of dignity of his position, and as the Prince, so oddly named Siegfried, Robert Helpmann has that supreme artistry that makes even the nebulous hero of classical ballet seem a living and moving character, sensitively realised down to so small a detail as the little sudden smile with which he makes the flight of swans overhead vivid to the audience. His acting in the third Act, in which the Prince can so easily seem a purely lay figure, is an exercise in subtlety and restraint in which the smallest movement is revealing. Helpmann can give his dancing considerable strength when he feels the character, as in *Job* and *The Wanderer*, demands it; here he combines princeliness with grace, and chooses a poetic interpretation of a Prince whose romantic imagination could only be touched by the figure, half-bird, half-woman, of a dolorous and enchanted princess. When he is below his best form his dancing of the third Act variation lacks something of the diamond-crisp attack of Petipa classicism, the one moment in the ballet when it is required and which he magnificently achieves in his partnering in the *Sleeping Beauty* and *Casse Noisette adagios;* but at all times he has the long, pure leg-line, the beautifully arched *point tendu* and litheness of limb of the true *danseur noble*, together with phenomenal balance in an arabesque pose. His third Act *jetés* have a winged excitement and his partnering is in the impeccable *danseur noble* tradition of musicianship and tact which no other English dancer since Dolin seems to have been able to reproduce.

The pivot of this ballet, however, must always be the ballerina, and Margot Fonteyn dominates the action both in that ease that comes of technical mastery as well as the innate dignity of the *prima ballerina*. That she possesses the qualities that distinguish the artist from the mere technician is apparent in her Swan Princess, to which she gives a moonlit radiance, softness and pathos without impairing her regality or the cool purity and extension of her classical "line." Her Odette excels above all in its poetry, its sense of flight exquisitely conveyed in hands and arms, its slow, smooth unfolding of the leg in a perfectly poised arabesque like a spreading wing. Like Helpmann she acts with heart and mind, and nothing in this performance is more characteristic, and more moving, than her pitying glance at the departing swans before she too is irresistibly drawn back into bondage; she and they in that moment become linked in a common disaster. Fonteyn is too much an artist to appear at her best in the pure acrobatics of the third Act *fouettés*, but her attack, pride and gaily-veiled malevolence are here in sufficient contrast to the lyricism of her Odette, and her dancing has speed and a strong, clear "line."

Beryl Grey, sixteen years of age at the time of this revival, had already proved herself an Odette-Odile of brilliant promise. A classical dancer of fluent technique and musicality, her Odette was sweet if immature, and she effectively brought to the wicked Odile something of the seductive vitality of her Duessa. In later performances she has gained both in depth and sweep of movement, and at her best she has a marble quality of "line" that suggests the complete ballerina, although her height tends to be a handicap in supported work and she lacks the advantage Fonteyn had from an early age of Helpmann's assured and selfless partnering. Pamela May after her return to the company also danced the parts with increasing speed and control, the last particularly noticeable in the fine balance of her slow pirouettes *en attitude* in the third Act variation. As Odette her accent on tragic queenliness provided an interesting contrast to Margot Fonteyn's lyrical tenderness, for her classicism, like that of Danilova, is cold rather than romantic, but her performances suggested she had still to acquire the mental discipline that can cover the physical strain of dancing a four-Act ballet. During 1944 Moira Shearer also danced the third Act with the resilient poise of the ballerina and a bright, burnished beauty that made the audience gasp. Her acting was excellent and this was an important step forward in the career of a young dancer, then seventeen years old, who showed she had every natural gift of the ballerina. Certainly she is an Odette-Odile of future distinction.

John Hart, before he joined the Royal Air Force, danced and partnered extremely well in the part of the Prince, and David Paltenghi, though lacking the technique and "line" of the classical dancer, afterwards worked hard at a part he would not normally have been called upon to dance and carried it off by reason of his intelligent acting, good partnering and stage presence. The ratio of performances of *Lac des Cygnes* by Fonteyn and Helpmann—approximately one in four—was not high enough in the latter part of the war to keep the interpretation of this ballet on a consistent artistic level; the "star" system has its disadvantages, but in the theatre the front-rank talent cannot and should not be prevented from emerging, and the dependence of classical ballet on the dancer is such that if standards are to be maintained it must be performed by the finest and most mature artists more regularly than by any others, even if this means less frequent performance of the ballet concerned. It is the recognition of this truth in Russia, together with a magnificently-graded system of training of the dancers, that has kept the classical tradition from disintegration and the standard of performance higher, all competent observers appear to agree, than anywhere in the world.

THE SLEEPING BEAUTY

THE original Sadler's Wells production of this ballet, performed like the Diaghileff production of 1921 under the title of *The Sleeping Princess*, disappeared from the repertoire in 1942 after a period of obvious disintegration due partly to the male call-up and the youth and inexperience of the company at that time. It was felt also that the staging was inadequate in view of the company's growing scale of achievement in its production of modern works, and it was planned not to revive the ballet until new scenery and costumes could be designed by Oliver Messel, whose ravishingly beautiful designs for the Old Vic "Romantic period" production of *A Midsummer Night's Dream*, including a succession of flower-embossed gauze curtains, had been in the full tradition of the "transformation scene" ballet of which *The Sleeping Beauty* is the finest extant example.

With its beautiful Tchaikovsky score, its magnificent Rose and fourth-Act *adagios*, its Blue Bird variations and fine contrast of peasant, Court and classic dancing in the third Act, this ballet is, however, a touchstone of Petipa choreography and the repertoire cannot be considered complete without it. For all its defects of *décor* and performance the earlier Wells production brought an electric current of anticipation into the auditorium that no other ballet could evoke, and there is no doubt this was principally due to Margot Fonteyn's Princess Aurora, the most radiant and authoritative of her performances and the one in which she most truly attained the grandeur and breadth of style of the Petipa ballerina. Her equilibrium in the Rose *adagio* was faultless, and when she and Helpmann as her Prince, dazzling in white bridal satin, stepped on to the stage for the great *pas de deux* it was as if the spirit of classicism had taken body and shape. Helpmann's Prince, especially in the Vision scene with its long passages of mime, had exceptional magnetism in gesture and the creation of atmosphere, his *pirouettes à la seconde* in his variation were notable for their finesse and his and Fonteyn's performance of the fourth Act *adagio*, the most spectacular and exciting of all classical *pas de deux*, set a standard in execution and partnering all balletgoers and dancers should have constantly in mind. He later enlivened the production with a ghoulish and fantastically old-womanish portrait of the wicked Fairy Carabosse, the part created by Enrico Cecchetti (who also danced the Blue Bird) in the original St. Petersburg production.

Harold Turner and Mary Honer danced the Blue Birds in this first production with glittering *élan*, and June Brae, glowing in personality and a mime of true artistry, played the Lilac Fairy. The six difficult and beautiful Fairy variations of the Prologue never came off *in toto*, but Margaret Dale's Fairy of the Song Birds and Julia Farron's meticulous "finger" variation were constant factors of a very high standard, and when Beryl Grey, with her spectacular arabesque, appeared as the Camellia Fairy one had an exciting glimpse of true classical style.

The reopening of Covent Garden Opera House on 20th February 1946 with a performance of this ballet crowned fifteen years' fine and increasing achievement by the Sadler's Wells company under the direction of Ninette de Valois. With this appearance at a theatre of great ballet traditions English ballet came to full maturity, and the effect on the dancers was apparent in a performance which surpassed any of their previous ones in classical breadth, vitality and finish.

It is significant of the basic policy of this company that the management chose to mark this great occasion in its history by a performance of a Russian classical ballet and not of ballets representing its own considerable choreographic achievement. Always recognising the importance of the classical tradition as a' foundation stone of modern dancing and choreography, Miss de Valois in this production was able to show the high technical level her dancers had now reached, and through them the justification of her policy. This was not only a brilliant and exciting occasion in itself, it was a herald of the achievement that might be expected of English dancers in their own creative ballets in the future. For "in order to dance the new ballets successfully," as Pavlova has said, "it is indispensable to have passed through a school of classical dancing."

It is the choreography of Petipa above all that represents the classical dance in its most refined expression. The construction of his great four-Act ballets, with their scenes of *divertissement* alternating with passages of mime, may be outmoded by modern standards, but their emphasis on visual qualities of line and grace and virtuosity of movement remain unequalled, a necessary education for dancers, choreographers and audience alike. In *corps de ballet* arrangement, though excellently inventive at his best, he had his moments when routine outpaced inspiration, and even in Russia it is customary to rearrange his choreography from time to time. There was therefore full precedent for the rechoreographing of the Garland Waltz by Frederick Ashton for this production, and he has done this with inventiveness and charm. The arrangements in the last Act were less happy. As in the Diaghileff version the Diamond, Gold, Silver and Sapphire Fairies were replaced by the dance "Florestan and his Sisters," again choreographed by Ashton but less well than in the case of the Waltz. Moira Shearer and Gerd Larsen danced their variations with precise and sparkling classic style, but the male solo (perhaps partly because the music was written for a woman) was weak and the Coda set an ugly and impossible task for the dancers. The omission of the Prince's solo and classical Coda from the choreography for Aurora and the Prince, and the substitution of the character dance, the Three Ivans, between the great *adagio* and Aurora's solo, was also an odd arrangement that badly broke the classical sequence and made the exquisite little variation for Aurora, danced by Margot Fonteyn with brilliant crispness and delicacy of hand movements, seem an anti-climax.

The rearrangements were the more unfortunate since they accentuated the weakness of the male situation, a continuing legacy of the war years. The Three Ivans demands a *brio* in execution outside the range of English dancers (Harold Turner and Gordon Hamilton, both Russian trained, proved notable exceptions), and the omission of the Prince's solo left Helpmann with no dancing except in the second Act Court dance, where his perfectly-controlled slow pirouettes were a delight for the *connoisseur*. Alexis Rassine at his best has given sparkle and a new fluid control to the male Blue Bird and once again proved himself the best classical dancer, after Helpmann, in a company not strong on the male side and not always ready to make use of its best.

With the absence of *The Sleeping Beauty* from the repertoire, as well as the lack of opportunity to dance regularly on a large stage, Margot Fonteyn inevitably lost a fraction of the *brio* and breadth of style that are hers by heritage and artistic progression; but her performance always stood as an illumination of her true possibilities as a ballerina, and the Covent Garden revival was memorable for her splendid re-adjustment of personality and style to suit the magnitude of stage and auditorium. Always an enchanting Aurora, she has never danced with such fire and beauty, and combined ease, grace and speed of movement with such breathtaking balance and extension of "line." She has, moreover, a full sense of the character in all its phases; light and gay as morning sunlight in the first Act, she has in the Vision scene something of the elusive shimmer of stars reflected in moving water, and attains in the last the shining nobility and spaciousness of

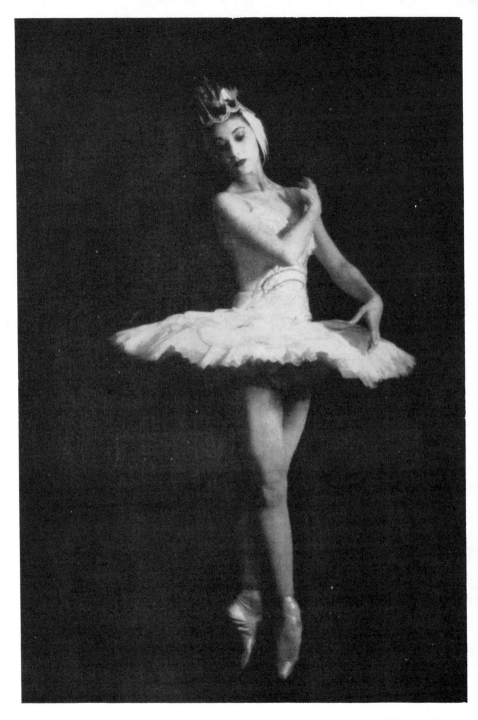

Photo

Le Lac des Cygnes
Margot Fonteyn as Odette

Tunbridge-Sedgwick

Plate XXXVII

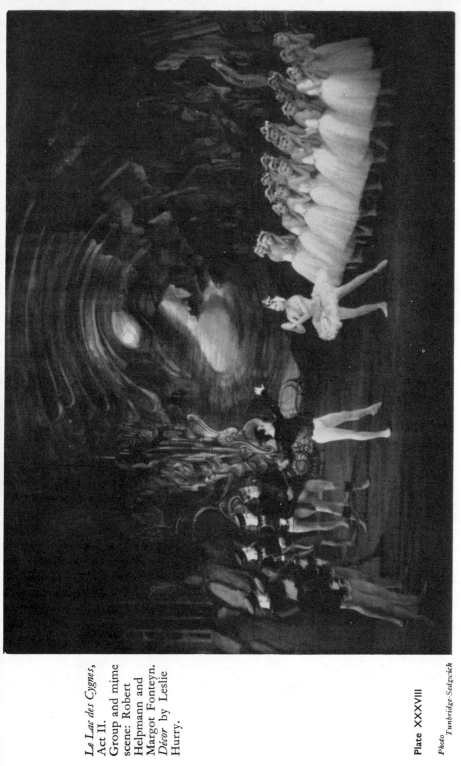

Le Lac des Cygnes,
Act II.
Group and mime
scene: Robert
Helpmann and
Margot Fonteyn.
Décor by Leslie
Hurry.

Plate XXXVIII

Photo Tunbridge-Sedgwick

Plate XXXIX

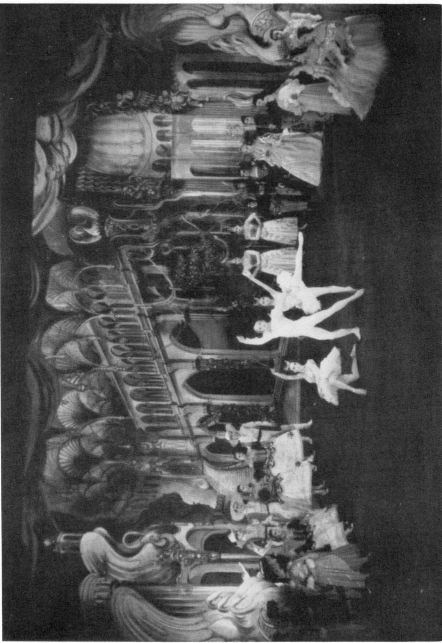

Le Lac des Cygnes, Act III. Pas de Trois: Joan Sheldon, Alexis Rassine and Margaret Dale. *Décor* by Leslie Hurry

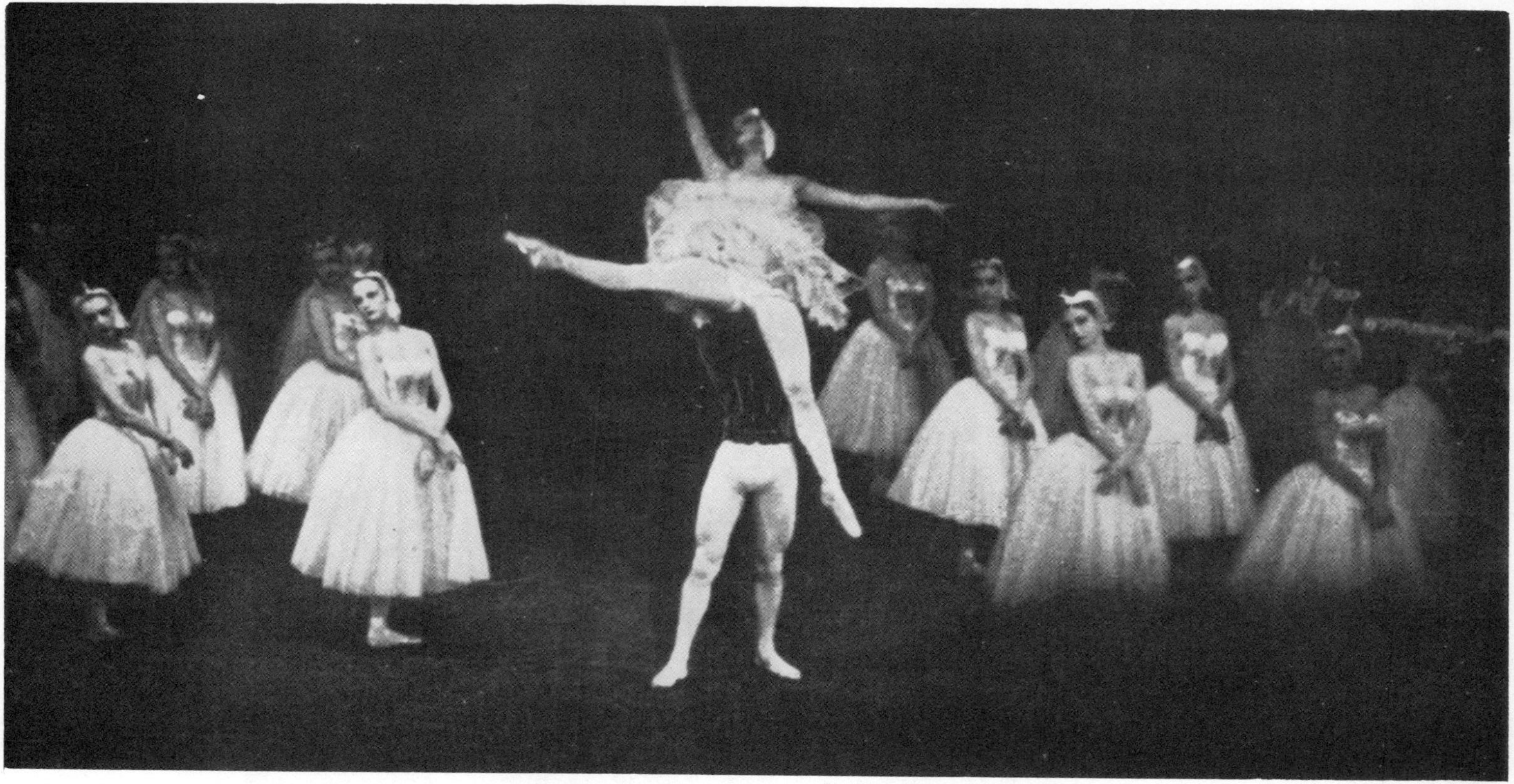

Action Photo G. B. L. *Wilson*

Plate XL

Le Lac des Cygnes. Act II: "Lift" in Pas de Deux: Beryl Grey

Action Photo

G. B. L. Wilson

Giselle, Act II. Pas de Deux: Margot Fonteyn and Robert Helpmann

Plate XII

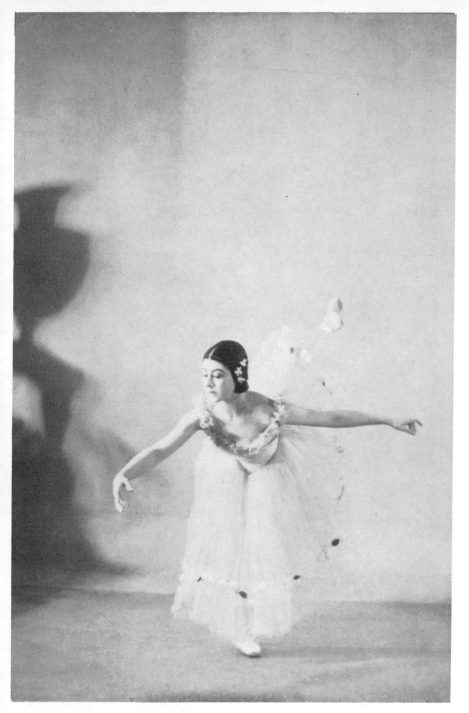

Giselle
Margot Fonteyn as Giselle

Plate XLII

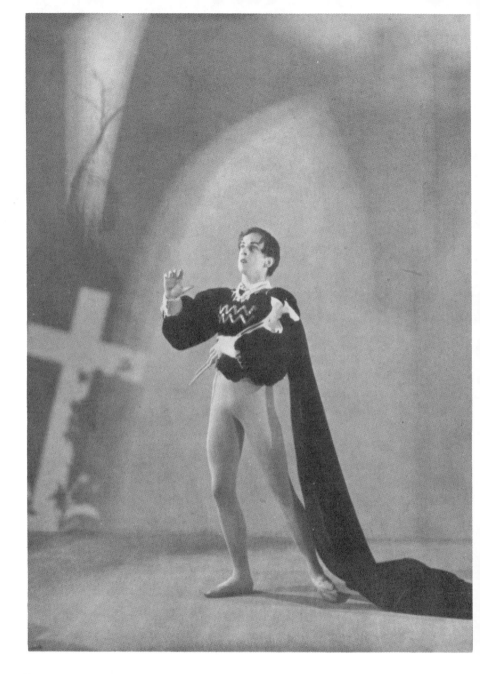

Giselle
Robert Helpmann as Albrecht

Plate XLIII

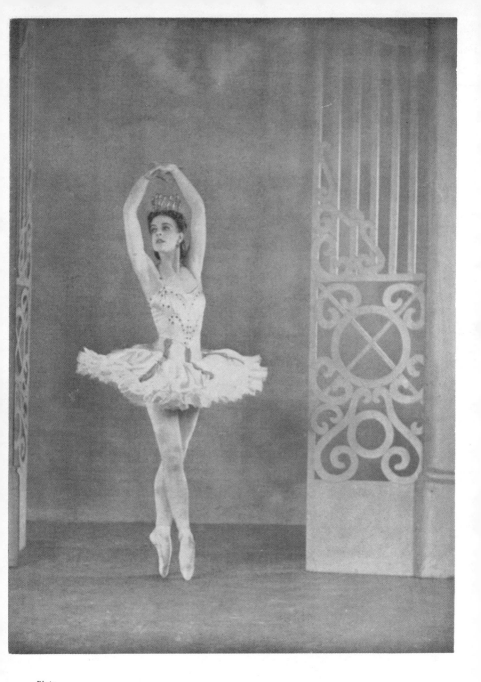

Photo

Anthony

Casse Noisette
Pamela May as the Sugar Plum Fairy

Plate XLIV

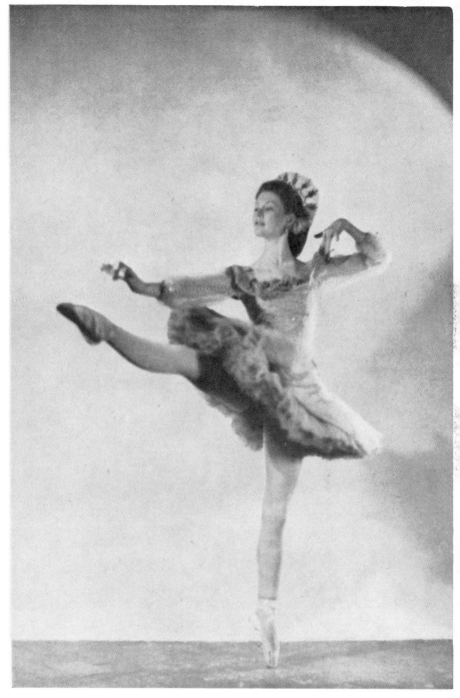

Photo
Anthony

The Sleeping Beauty
The Rose Adagio: Moira Shearer as Aurora

Plate XLV

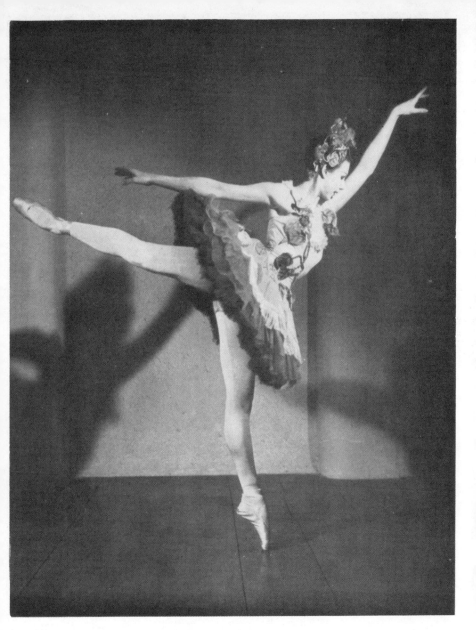

The Sleeping Beauty
Beryl Grey as the Lilac Fairy

Plate XLVI

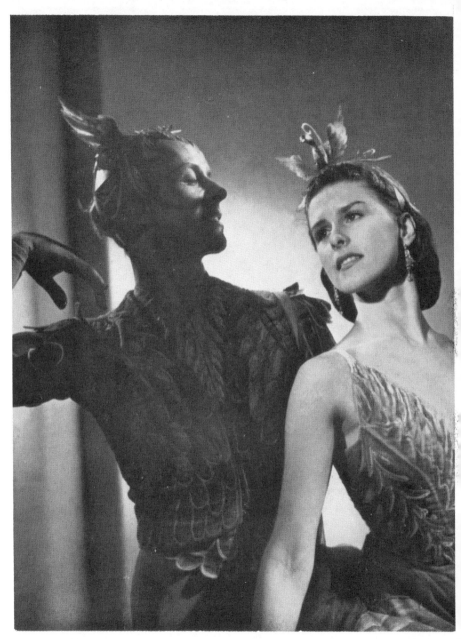

The Sleeping Beauty
Harold Turner and Violetta Prokhorova as the Blue Birds

Plate XLVII

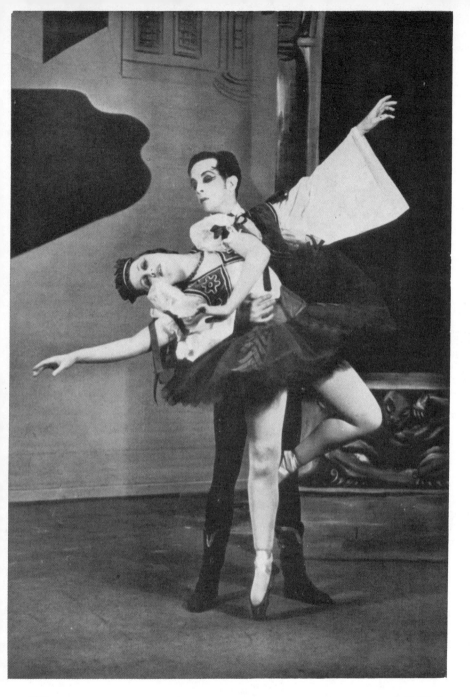

Photo
J. W. Debenham

Coppélia
Swanhilda and Franz: Mary Honer and Robert Helpmann

Plate XLVIII

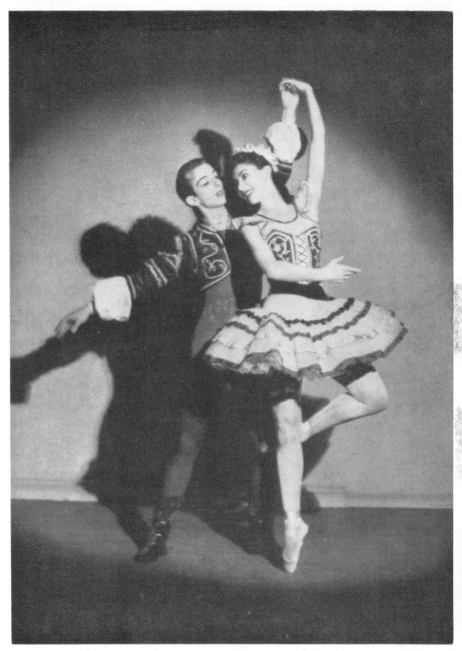

Coppélia
Swanhilda and Franz: Margot Fonteyn and Alexis Rassine

Plate XLIX

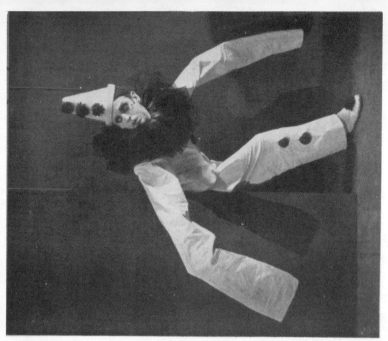

Edward Mandinian

Carnaval
Robert Helpmann as Pierrot

Plate LI

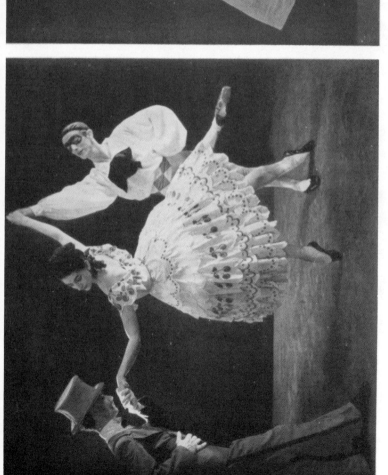

Photos

Carnaval
Gordon Hamilton (Pantalon), Margot Fonteyn (Columbine) and
Alexis Rassine (Harlequin)

Plate L

Photo
Edward Mandinian

Plate LII

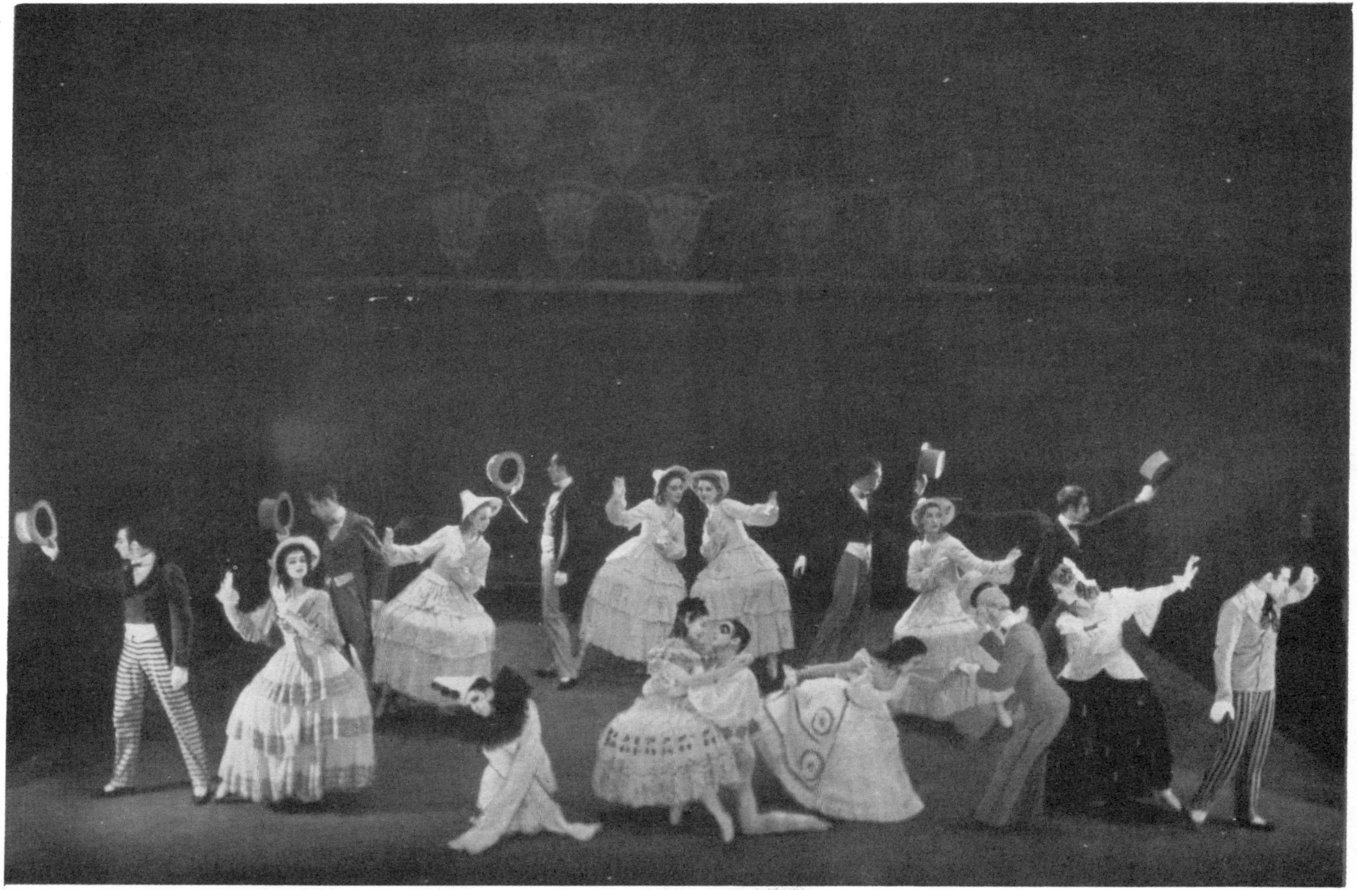

Carnaval.
Final group:
Sadler's Wells
Ballet.

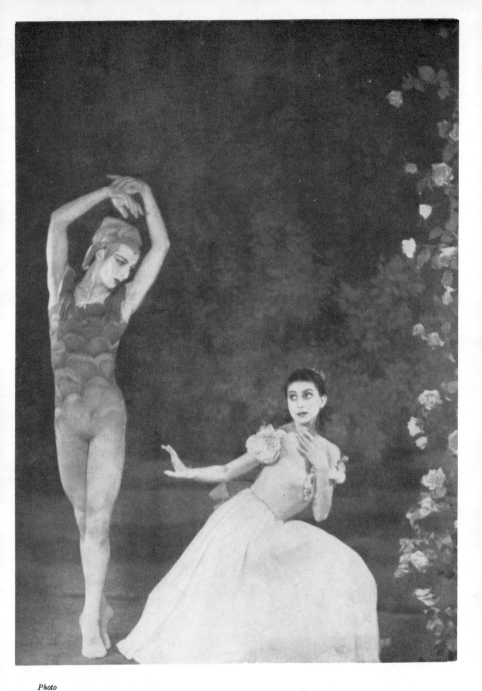

Le Spectre de la Rose
Alexis Rassine and Margot Fonteyn

Plate LIII

movement of the true ballet Princess. This is a great ballerina performance by any standards. As before she is finely supported by Robert
Helpmann, who mimes the Prince with his incomparable sensitivity
and clarity of gesture and romantic insight, and on the First Night
played the wicked Fairy Carabosse with a malevolent grandeur,
tinged with sardonic humour, that "lifted" the performance practically
out of the theatre and into the Market outside. Covent Garden even
is scarcely big enough for this personality.

Moira Shearer's elegance of style, Anne Negus's musicality and
smoothness in *pas de bourrée*, Margaret Dale's razor-sharp attack,
Gillian Lynne's fluid unfolding of arabesque and Beryl Grey's
extended "line" and radiant presence as the Fairy of the Lilac, were
valuable in a series of dances, the Fairy variations, which exploit to
the full both the variety of Petipa's invention and Tchaikovsky's
command of melody and rhythm. In addition to her outstanding
"finger" variation Margaret Dale also gave to the White Cat a proud
and amusing touch of the *ballerina assoluta*, and later danced the
Blue Bird with a fluttering swiftness. It was in the part of the Blue
Bird, on the second night of this revival, that the young Moscow
dancer, Violetta Prokhorova, made her first appearance in this country.
Technically Prokhorova is not stronger than several English dancers;
but though her arm movements are unorthodox they have a noble
sweep and flow, and of her it can truly be said she dances with every
part of her body. With her fabulous instep and *développé* and sunlit
charm Prokhorova brought a new and vital aspect of Russian
classicism to the English stage.

Not all later performances have been of high standard, especially
in the case of the leading fairies, where it is absolutely essential the
dancers should have ballerina "line" and presence for the supported
work as well as the technique for the solos. It would be idle also to
pretend that the company possesses another ballerina of Margot
Fonteyn's status for the rôle of Aurora. Pamela May, however, has
danced the part with a new lyrical fluency and attained real authority
in the supported *adagio* work, although her Vision scene tended to
be earthbound and one was conscious occasionally of a lack of stamina
for so exacting a rôle. Moira Shearer, dancing here her first full-length
ballerina rôle, gave encouraging proof of staying power and apart
from slight faults of inexperience this was, even from the beginning,
a performance of crystal-clear technique, poise and beauty. Her
Russian training is apparent in the way this dancer takes the stage

and her Vision scene has a translucent expressiveness and grace. David Paltenghi as the Prince supported both these Auroras very well, but classical ballet really needs a more highly trained *danseur noble* with the "line," attack and speed of movement which alone can enhance the exciting quality of the ballerina in a *pas de deux*. Gordon Hamilton's Carabosse, witch-like after Helpmann's subtle and flashing Spanish *grande dame*, had a fine sense of gesture and the *corps de ballet* danced well throughout, although more uniformity and grace of head and arm position would add to the style of English dancing generally. There is a need, too, for more personality and joy of movement.

The revival was staged with a magnificence not surpassed by Russian Ballet performances in this country. The cumbersome costumes for the Waltz mask the pattern of the dance just as Margot Fonteyn's headdress in Act I tends to cut the line of her neck; but the beauty and fantasy of Oliver Messel's designs generally, and the classic spaciousness of his settings, with their vistas of Versailles fountains and marble staircases, capture the atmosphere and enchantment of the fairy tale. His ruby-red velvet hunting costume for the Prince, recalling an eighteenth-century French Marquis, is the finest in the ballet; that for the same character in the last Act, with its oppressive coronet, the least successful. The excellent new orchestra, under Constant Lambert, gave full richness and glow to Tchaikovsky's score, and prepared us for a brilliant *entr'acte* rendering, later in the first Covent Garden season, of Alan Rawsthorne's fine fantasy-overture, *Cortèges*.

CASSE NOISETTE

THE last Act of *The Sleeping Beauty*, with its fairy-tale atmosphere and superb *adagios* and variations, is so superior to the last-Act *divertissement* of *Casse Noisette* that it is strange that it has not similarly been used in England as a separate item on the programme. (The Diaghileff *divertissement* entitled *Aurora's Wedding*, which is all that survives of *The Sleeping Beauty* in Russian-American companies, is actually a selection of dances from both ballets, with some interpolated numbers by Nijinska. It serves to provide both dancers and audience with a living experience in Petipa classicism but the difference in quality between the two scores—for Tchaikovsky himself, uninspired by the scenario, considered *Casse Noisette* one of his poorer works—detracts from any value it might possess as an artistic entity.) The first scene of *Casse Noisette*, when played, has the charm of a Russian

Christmas party for children but small dancing interest. The early Wells performances of the ballet, in which Markova danced the Sugar Plum Fairy with scintillating delicacy and Robert Helpmann, when not taking his turn with Harold Turner as her cavalier, gave a lively oddity to a Chinaman with Walter Gore, had a glint of magic that tended to vanish later, although in the revivals Margot Fonteyn has brought to the *adagio* something of the resplendent erectness and nobility of "line" of her Princess Aurora. Pamela May, with her sun-bright beauty and high, clean *developpé* and arabesque, has also danced this part with a strong measure of assurance, giving the *adagio* more the quality of a love duet than any other dancer. Helpmann's variation in this ballet, light and flawless in balance, is perhaps his finest individual piece of classical dancing. The attractive variations of the *Valse des Fleurs*, the only other classical dances of interest in the ballet, have been executed with consistent fluidity and style, but the Dance of the Mirletons, in which the turned-out positions are so exaggerated that the dancers come perilously near to turning themselves inside out, is an illuminating example of the trite and uglier form of classicism against which Fokine, the poet of the dance, revolted.

COPPÉLIA

MARGOT FONTEYN'S London début as Swanhilda in *Coppélia*, on 25th January 1943, gave a glitter of excitement to a New Theatre first night and put this seventy-year-old classical ballet into a "star" place in the repertoire it had not held since Adeline Genée danced it at the old Empire. *Coppélia* is one of the most charming of the doll ballets. It has neither the compact artistry nor the satiric sense of character of *Boutique Fantasque*, and the choreography lacks that touch of sensibility that makes Massine's Can-Can Dancers suddenly moving. But it has fun and verve, a delicious score, and a part for the ballerina which is technically one of the most brilliant in all ballet. Margot Fonteyn tackled it with a speed and lightness that were remarkable when one considered how overworked she had been at this time, and that her pointwork has an acquired rather than a natural hardness. Her second-Act arabesque *en tournant* has a clear-cut height and smoothness and her gaiety and mimic invention in this part show a marked widening of dramatic range. The performance has the sparkle of champagne, and if bubbling high spirits and a sense of fun are substituted for the more usual *soubrette* piquancy, why not? No part, from Hamlet downwards, can be nailed down to one interpretation, and the great artist will give to all rôles a touch of individuality. Fonteyn's Swanhilda is not in the least like that of Mary Honer, her predecessor in the part, who gave it a saucer-eyed wistfulness and mischief and a steel-pointed technique of glittering virtuosity; but its lighter and more purely classical elegance is equally enchanting, and in responsiveness and wit it keeps the scenes with Dr. Coppelius on a high level of spontaneous humour.

The same question of difference of interpretation (for the ballet outlook is, in the main, a conservative one) has occurred in respect of Robert Helpmann's Dr. Coppelius, a part many people seem to believe in all seriousness "was not meant to be funny." The truth is there is no set tradition attached to this part at all, as a famous ballerina found when she danced in the ballet in a succession of Continental cities with a Dr. Coppelius that varied, according to the district, from an elegant aristocrat in powdered wig to a comic butt. Helpmann plays it with a crusty sense of caricature and comic invention, together with that touch of pathos—in the old man's breathless, awed delight when the doll comes to life, his grief and disappointment when he realises the trick—that one finds in the work of all great clowns. A richly-embroidered and unforced piece of pantomime, it has a Dickensian instinct for idiosyncrasy and has brought the comedy to life in a way no other recent performance has succeeded in doing.

The witty subtleties of mime which Helpmann previously contrived to bring to the romantic part of Franz disappeared when he gave up the rôle; but John Hart has danced it with refreshing spirit and style and Alexis Rassine, miming here with a lively charm, has given the third-Act variation a flight-like grace and clarity of "line." Rassine's partnering is not strong and he is not always completely finished, but he is a born classical dancer who has been of considerable value to the company during a difficult period. The standard of performance of this ballet by the Sadler's Wells company is generally high; even in the depredations of war-time the first-Act Mazurka and Czardas have retained an excellent degree of zest, and the variations of Swanhilda and her six friends, with Délibes's orchestration at its most complex and rhythmic, are gay and clear. The choreography of the first two Acts is inventive and firm in outline, an exercise in classical execution, and the *pas de deux* with the ear of corn in the first scene and Swanhilda's Spanish dance and Scotch reel, neatly adapted to classic technique, in the second are expertly arranged to exploit the dancer's "line" and control in *adagio* and volatility in *allegro*. The version danced by

Sadler's Wells is based on that produced by Ivanov and Cecchetti in Russia and probably little of the original choreography of Saint-Léon remains. William Chappell's costumes and scenery had a tuppence-coloured prettiness that added immeasurably to the bright inconsequence of the ballet, and Peggy Van Praagh, though not a classical dancer in "line," has also danced Swanhilda with attractive personality and technical pace. Pamela May, a true classicist in physique and arabesque, is a more recent addition to a distinguished line of Sadler's Wells Swanhildas beginning with Lydia Lopokova.

Margot Fonteyn has now danced all five of the great classical rôles, and in perfection of build, intelligence and effortlessness of technique she belongs to the purest type of classical *danseuse*. She has progressed steadily in range and expression, and her hands and arms, pliant, unaffected and continuing her leg extension in a lovely unbroken line, she has developed, after some initial untidiness, into an indivisible part of her dance. In this she is a model to English dancers, who tend to break the line which in Russian classicism flows gracefully from wrist to ankle and to mar their style by stiff arms, bent elbows and spreading fingers. Possibly Fonteyn is still not at the height of her powers but that she has been able to progress at all under the gruelling conditions of performance in war-time is a tribute to her powers of assimilation and will to work. On the classical side her influence has been as important as that of Helpmann in modern ballet; it is principally owing to her dancing that English ballet has been able to maintain the classical ballets in the repertoire with anything of their native brilliance, and the maintenance of such ballets is of the utmost importance in the education not only of dancers but of audience.

The lack of classical standards in the past in America was mainly due to the fact that the second Act of *Lac des Cygnes* and the *Aurora's Wedding divertissement*, in brief visits by the Diaghileff and de Basil companies (no American city until recently proved capable of supporting more than one week of ballet at a stretch) were the only examples of pure classicism seen there in a performance of high professional standard. As a result the free dance movement took root in a way it was never able to do in England, where classical traditions were more firmly grounded. The revival of the Russian classical ballets by the Sadler's Wells company in their entirety has played a leading part in consolidating that tradition in England, and it is mainly through the dancing of the first Sadler's Wells ballerina, Alicia Markova, that classicism is at last taking root in America, although full-length productions of *Lac des Cygnes* and *The Sleeping Beauty* can still only be seen, on isolated annual occasions, in the repertoire of the San Francisco Ballet.

CHAPTER XV

FOKINE AND THE ENGLISH BALLET

LES SYLPHIDES

FOKINE is the only modern choreographer whose ballets have already become classics in the sense that they appear in the repertoire of every world company, and in England his romantic works take their place beside the earlier Russian classics as a valuable contribution to general choreographic and dancing standards. In essence and intention representing a revolt against the more rigid conventions of Petipa classicism, they more directly derive in style from the romanticism of *Giselle* than from *The Sleeping Beauty;* but now thirty years have passed it is possible to see how completely Fokine built on the classical groundwork of his immediate predecessors. The mental approach was different, but the technique, although softened and lyricised, was essentially the same, and *Les Sylphides* to-day is nearer to pure classicism than most of the ballets of the outstanding modern choreographers.

Les Sylphides, the abstract ballet *par excellence* and in the construction of pure dance patterns Fokine's masterpiece, is a work that demands, for its true effect, a complete assimilation of the romantic spirit in its dancers. "Isadora Duncan," wrote Prince Peter Lieven, "was the first to bring out in her dancing the meaning of the music; she was the first to *dance* the music and not dance *to* the music. She altered the whole direction of the dance from pure movement to movement expressing sound." Although this is probably an overstatement, since the introduction into ballet of composers of the rank of Tchaikovsky and Glazunov had already had some effect in the encouragement of musical expressiveness in choreographers and dancers, it is true in the sense that Isadora Duncan was the first to create and dance with a full consciousness of the musical revolution she was directing and inspiring.

Les Sylphides is the classical consummation of this ideal; it is from first to last a reflection of the rhythm, feeling and melodic outline of

Chopin's music, and the dancers, like the dances they interpret, must drift with the music as if it were an inborn part of them. Nowhere is this more necessary than in the "lifts" in the Grand Valse; the dancer here must seem as light as a snowflake, rising, floating and descending on the surface of the musical line. It is an effect that depends on the musical ear of the partner as well as on the grace and spirituality of the dancer herself, and it is Robert Helpmann's extraordinary musicality as well as his natural romanticism which has made him the best male Sylphide of his generation. He is almost alone among dancers, as Paderewski was among pianists, to reflect the subtle and elusive *tempo rubato* of Chopin's music, and his omission for a period of several years from the Sadler's Wells cast was a very grave mistake. His return has provided the necessary foil to Margot Fonteyn's limpid flowing technique and poetry of expression. As in *Giselle* Fonteyn covers her lack of elevation in the Mazurka with the remote beauty of her dance, and her arabesques, softly extended, have the sense of spiritualised yearning Fokine himself aimed at expressing through this pure classical movement. Celia Franca, with her beautiful suppleness of hands and arms and feeling for musical phrasing, has extracted the true essence of the Prelude, a dance in which Tatiana Riabouchinska set a standard of sensibility and which Margot Fonteyn, with her indefinable musicality, would also perform to perfection. Moira Shearer's cool, grave beauty of arabesque and Anne Negus's finesse and rhythmic subtlety in the Waltz, one of the loveliest of Fokine's inventions, have also been notable, the last dancer displaying a skimming swiftness and evenness in the *pas de bourrées* of the *finale* that revive something of the delicate art of a step that seems to evade modern dancers.

With dancers such as these, the original Benois backcloth, and a *corps de ballet* which at its best preserves the spirit and pattern of the dances, the Sadler's Wells company is capable of that rarity in ballet performance, a really good *Sylphides;* unfortunately frequent change of cast rarely allows the ballet to be seen with a complete team of front-rank soloists, and this production needed softer or dimmer lighting and the more usual little starry wreaths of flowers in the dancers' hair to give it pictorial as well as spiritual atmosphere. Beryl Grey has been most successful in this company after Fonteyn in capturing the lyrical grace of the Grand Valse and the Mazurka; although the first has been exquisitely performed, with perfect elegance of style, by Sally Gilmour of the Ballet Rambert and in the Anglo-

Polish Ballet Hélène Wolska, an English dancer of considerable virtuosity who was a pupil and discovery of Nijinska, has given to both dances that insubstantiality and *ballon*, the quality of floating on air, that is in the direct line of artistic heritage from Taglioni and Pavlova. *Les Sylphides* has the very texture of gossamer, it is all spirit, and its only flaw in construction is the long and rather jarring break in the action just before the end when the dancers return to the empty stage to take up their positions for the final Grand Valse.

LE SPECTRE DE LA ROSE

THE fragile and air-spun fantasy of *Le Spectre de la Rose* has eluded recapture almost continually since its first production, when Karsavina as the Young Girl and Nijinsky as the Spirit of the Rose created a legend of pure romance no subsequent dancers have been able to dispel. Baronova has charmingly caught at the poignancy, and Ruth Chanova the dreaming quality, of the part of the Young Girl, but neither of them had very sensitive support and the part of the Spirit of the Rose, which in Nijinsky's performance is said to have had a spiritual magic that transcended mere technique, has long since degenerated to athleticism.

In the Sadler's Wells production sensitively revived by Tamara Karsavina in 1944 it was possible to feel once again an intangible sympathy between the Girl and the spirit of her dream, and the imaginative beauty of Fokine's choreography for the Rose, with its gliding *pas de bourrées* and soft, weaving arm movements, was revealed by Karsavina with a new understanding. Though without a prodigious elevation, Alexis Rassine took to the air as if it were his natural element and used his arms with a flowing grace. A beautifully-built and supple dancer, this young Russian's success was at first hampered by what appeared to be a purely physical approach to his work; later he seems to have responded to his surroundings, in a company in which the dramatic values have always been emphasised as much as the technical, and his dancing in *Le Spectre de la Rose* showed, under Karsavina's guidance, a growing artistry. Never quite of the earth, with drooping eyelids that echoed the mood of sleep, this Spirit awakened the Girl with a *fey* protectiveness, and although the performance lacked the poetry and lightness that Helpmann would have brought to the part, and Turner's rather acrobatic swiftness and finish, it was more truly romantic in style than any of recent years. There were no reserves at all about Margot Fonteyn's performance of the Young Girl; this was enchanting, and her wonder, delight and regret mirrored the pathos of the unattainable. It was her acting, more than Rassine's dancing, that gave to the Rose an ethereal quality, and to the whole ballet the wistful evanescence of a vision. The part was later danced by Moira Shearer with a sleepy grace and a little pang of disappointment, on waking, that caught at the heart; but in the pure poetry of this ballet Pamela May has been less successful, her emotional maturity, which makes her outstanding in *Dante Sonata*, suggesting here a sophistication which is entirely lacking from Fonteyn's radiant and romance-enchanted Young Girl.

Le Spectre de la Rose, suggested to the poet Vaudoyer by a line in a poem by Gautier, is, like *Les Sylphides*, a posthumous tribute to the spirit of the Romantic movement in ballet. Composed to the music of Weber's *Invitation to the Waltz*, it was tossed off by Fokine in a few days as a stop-gap in the Diaghileff programmes; a brilliant improvisation that has outlasted many more ambitious works. Like *Les Sylphides* it is dependent to a large degree on atmosphere in production and performance, and in the case of the Sadler's Wells revival this was caught not only by the dancers but by the designer. Rex Whistler replaced Bakst's virginal white bedroom with one of equal charm in delicate ice-blue, and through two open french windows a moonlit garden and trailing roses, exquisitely painted, suggested the mysterious fragrance of a summer night. The "austerity" costume for the Rose was the one flaw.

Le Spectre de la Rose, following a splendid Romanesque *décor* for *Everyman* and a beautifully composed, classic-romantic backcloth for *Les Sylphides*, both war-time productions of the International Ballet, was Rex Whistler's last work for the theatre before he was killed in action in Normandy shortly after D-Day. He was serving as a lieutenant in the Welsh Guards, for which he had volunteered early in the war, and although it is in the nature of a digression I make no excuse for quoting intact, as a last tribute to one of the finest of modern ballet artists, the appreciation of his work which I wrote at the time of his death and which was published in *Theatre World* in September 1944:

> "The death of Rex Whistler on active service in Normandy has robbed the stage of a designer of unique and brilliantly adaptable period flair. Covering all styles from Rococo to Georgian, he yet retained an individuality and grace of line and colour that gave his work a vitality far transcending mere *pastiche*.

The Regency country house in *Pride and Prejudice*, the mid-Victorian palace in *Victoria Regina*, the drawing-room elegances of the nineties in *An Ideal Husband*, came sparklingly to life in his hands, and his work had a gay and fluent charm the stage can ill afford to lose.

"It is the tragedy of the scenic artist that his work is so ephemeral; producers when reviving plays look for fresh colours and backgrounds, and the surviving water-colour design on a neat but yellowed sheet of parchment, hung, if it is good enough, in an occasional 'Exhibition of Stage Design,' is an inadequate substitute for the three-dimensional spaciousness of the intended stage picture. Ballet, where the artist's contribution is an integral part of the whole, is a more lasting medium for the artist and it is through his ballets that Rex Whistler will probably be most remembered. *The Wise Virgins*, a Hebraic parable seen exquisitely through the eyes of the Italian Renaissance, and *The Rake's Progress*, in which the Hogarthian atmosphere of tawdriness and flamboyance was vigorously reproduced, are inconceivable without his settings and costumes, and in the C.E.M.A. Exhibition of Ballet Design last year his drawings for this last classic of English Ballet were outstanding in a room rich in the work of Benois, Bakst and Hurry. A fine draughtsman, with a magnificently clean architectural line and perspective, his drop curtain of an eighteenth-century London street for *The Rake's Progress* is, perhaps, the peak of his achievement in English Ballet. It is fitting that his last stage work, *Le Spectre de la Rose*, should also have been for the Sadler's Wells Ballet."

CARNAVAL

PERHAPS of all Fokine's ballets *Carnaval* is the one most dependent for its atmosphere on subtlety of interpretation, and an appreciation by the dancers of the pattern and style of the ballet as a whole. It is a balanced and stylised piece of machinery in which every cog should be as finely inter-related as Fokine's choreography and Bakst's designs are inter-related with Schumann's music. In the theme of this ballet, an imaginative expression of the spirit and period of the music, the mischief and gaiety of the *Commedia del 'Arte* are combined with the romance of an early Victorian ball, and although, apart from the essential sense of "style," most of the characters admit of more than one interpretation, perhaps the ideal performance is the one in which the dancers most successfully blend the glittering and the lyrical. There is wistfulness as well as lightness in Fokine's conception for those who will probe beneath its shining surface; in the sudden grave interlacing beauty of the dance of the three deserted girls, a serenely beautiful invention based on the *pas de bourrée*, in the tender charm of the entrance of Harlequin and Columbine, his arm protectively encircling her waist and his slow steps beating a contrapuntal measure beside her demure little run on full point, in the pale and woebegone figure of Pierrot, humour touched with pain, a Don Quixote whom romance eternally eludes.

It is because the dancers capture this lyrical and romantic undercurrent that the Sadler's Wells production of *Carnaval*, revived at the Princes Theatre in October 1944, seems to me preferable to some Russian performances I have seen of far more brilliant precision. The ensemble work is occasionally ragged, and not all of the *danseuses* have the necessary Dresden china daintiness and style; but the youthfulness, the gaiety and the mockery are without heartlessness, only the forlorn isolation of Pierrot, continually ignored and forgotten, carries a sting.

If this more English interpretation of the ballet differs from that of the Russian original (Cyril Beaumont[1] has referred to Karsavina's Columbine as "a heartless coquette" and to Nijinsky's Harlequin as "one lively as Mercury and maliciously mischievous as Tyl") it is perfectly in the spirit of Schumann's music and has its own charm. Margot Fonteyn as Columbine and Alexis Rassine as Harlequin were well matched in lightness and grace; there was warmth and sweetness in her happiness, and though his dancing was less faultless in finish and less musical than hers his gay, lithe fluency of movement was always attractive. The company has been happy in possessing three Chiarinas—Pamela May, Beryl Grey and Moira Shearer—of quite exceptional loveliness, elegance and grace, and Pauline Clayden's Papillon, radiant in white organdie, was well danced although it lacked the imponderable, airy flutter of the true butterfly. At later performances Papillon has been played by Anne Negus, an exquisitely danced interpretation with something of Kirsova's stylishness and glancing brilliance. Of the smaller parts Gordon Hamilton's elderly beau had a crisp and choleric humour and Julia Farron's Estrella had beautiful style. The key to the ballet, however, is Pierrot, though it is a key that has been lost in recent years when the part has become

[1] *The Diaghileff Ballet in London* (pub. Beaumont).

negligible or an exaggerated grotesque. Robert Helpmann played it, as it was played by its creator Adolph Bolm, as a figure of tragedy, with the result that the ballet gained that touch of humanity and pathos without which it tends to be a purely superficial flirtatious frolic. With a white face of haunting sadness and great black mournful dabs of eyes, Helpmann touched in the details with a gentle restraint and his little wry smile of resignation, when he realised the butterfly, like all his dreams, had escaped him, was movingly imagined.

The fresh, bright, paintbox colours of Bakst's *décor* and costumes have been reproduced in this production with care, and this is the only English revival in war-time which has caught the spirit and pattern of the ballet, although in the early productions of the International Ballet Harold Turner, supported with a charming mischief by Nina Tarakanova as Columbine, danced the part of Harlequin with the virtuosity only he, among English dancers, has been able at his best to give it.

These "trifles, light as air," are the only ballets of Fokine that have been seen in England in war-time; they express his romantic mood only, and until the return to England of Russian-trained companies after the war the strength and variety of the creator of the dramatic *Thamar*, the tragic *Petrouchka*, the pure Russian fantasy of *L'Oiseau de Feu*, will not become apparent to the vast new army of balletgoers which has sprung into being since 1939, when a Russian ballet company made its last appearance in England. The only version of the *Prince Igor* dances performed here during the war was not that of Fokine and the inferior choreography used has served only to emphasise how the genius of Fokine transformed his original material when he created the leaping and crossing lines, strong, fiery and barbaric, of his famous version of this opera ballet. The performance showed how completely Russian male character dancing of the national type is outside the range of an English company.

CHAPTER XVI

BALLET RAMBERT

MARIE RAMBERT can well claim to be the doyen of English ballet directors and since 1930, when the Ballet Rambert gave its first important season with Karsavina at the Lyric Theatre, Hammersmith, her organisation has provided a valuable training ground for English choreographers, designers and dancers, many of whom have since enriched the major companies of England and America. It was under her direct encouragement that Frederick Ashton, in 1926, created his first small ballet, *The Tragedy of Fashion*, a modernised version of the story, recounted by Madame de Sévigné, of the cook of Louis XIV who committed suicide because the fish was not delivered in time for the royal dinner party. This sophisticated satiric trifle, in which the cook was replaced by an up-to-date dress designer who killed himself with the scissors in passionate shame at the failure of one of his "creations," was presented in Nigel Playfair's production of *Riverside Nights*, with Marie Rambert and Ashton himself in the leading parts.

Antony Tudor and Andrée Howard among choreographers, Sophie Fedorovich, Nadia Benois, and William Chappell among designers, Harold Turner, Pearl Argyle, Maude Lloyd and, more recently, Sally Gilmour among dancers, are also in a large sense the discoveries of the Ballet Rambert, where they were given their earliest opportunities for artistic development. In the few years before the war this work was beginning to come to full fruition, the production of Tudor's *Jardin Aux Lilas* and *Dark Elegies*, and of Andrée Howard's *Lady Into Fox* and *Death and the Maiden*, giving the company a choreographic standard high enough to arrest attention in West End seasons. The secession of Anthony Tudor to form his own London Ballet in 1938 slightly weakened the company on the choreographic side, although during the "blitz" period of 1940, after Tudor's departure to America to take up the position of choreographer to the Ballet Theatre, the two companies amalgamated and presented non-stop programmes of ballet at the Arts Theatre throughout the worst of the bombing. Under such conditions, although some new work was presented, creative activity could hardly continue on as productive a scale as hitherto, and the enforced closing down of this prolific and adult little company for a period of two years, under a restrictive commercial contract, inevitably weakened the personnel.

When the Ballet Rambert was able to re-form and present a season at the Mercury Theatre, where it had had its first beginnings, in March 1944, the majority of its best dancers had migrated to other companies or been called into the Forces, and the task of building up afresh was hampered by the necessity of working once again on a tiny stage, and of undertaking long, courageous, but exhausting tours for C.E.M.A. in which it was necessary for the company to dance under a great variety of conditions in factories and provincial theatres. Yet soon the company began to find its feet again; both Sally Gilmour and Joan McClelland developed inconceivably as dancer-artists, and new choreographic work began to appear within a year of the Mercury Theatre season. In the summer of 1944 the company gave a further short season at the C.E.M.A.-controlled Lyric Theatre, Hammersmith, and the slightly larger stage enabled *Les Sylphides* and *Swan Lake*, Act II, to be given with a full *corps de ballet*. Presentation was still restricted by the lack of an orchestra and of a company of consistent dancing talent, but the Ballet School, with the Mercury Theatre as its headquarters, is in operation and the repertoire of revivals in this company's particular genre of *ballet intime* is a large one. At later London seasons an orchestra was added (although it proved more a liability than an asset at some performances), and a production of *Giselle*, Act II, with charming *décor* by Hugh Stevenson, was presented.

Frederick Ashton is the greatest choreographer this company can claim to have discovered and the most interesting aspect of the 1944 season was the opportunity given to see again some of his early works and trace the line of development to his recent ballets. I cannot look on *Les Masques*, for all its tart sophisticated invention, as anything but a side-step in Ashton's career; it shows very strongly the influence of his "revue" period and lacks the variety of wit and style that saves *Façade* from seeming equally ephemeral. *Capriol Suite*, however, produced three years earlier in the historic 1930 Hammersmith season, shows already the true Ashton and this little *suite de danses* leads in a direct choreographic line of succession to all his finest later work. It is full of the happiest and most lively invention, adapts folk dancing to stage technique with a subtle feeling for style, and captures the roistering as well as the lyrical and courtly aspects of the Elizabethan scene. All the dance springs naturally from Peter Warlock's enchanting suite of period airs, and the title of this gives the ballet a charming sentimental link with historic dance tradition; for Capriol was the name of the pupil in the dialogues which form the basis of the earliest French study of the dance, the *Orchésographie* of Thoinot Arbeau. This book, written by a priest with a passion for the art, was published in 1588 and the dances in Warlock's suite derive their names from the Court dances of the period described by Arbeau. *Capriol Suite*, which needs a small but good team of male dancers, has suffered from raggedness of execution in war-time performances, but the joyous floodtide of Ashton's invention, and the grave and lovely Pavane in which the red rose and scroll in the hands of the two male dancers suggest the amorous sweetness of the Elizabethan sonnet, have undimmed freshness and charm. Sara Luzita's languid Castilian beauty has been extraordinarily effective in this dance and *Capriol Suite* is still the best kind of Tudor-lore in this company. In *Mephisto Valse* one sees a further facet of Ashton's development, and his use of his dancers, even on the tiny Mercury stage, anticipates the growing mastery of *corps de ballet* pattern and accelerating excitement in *Apparitions* one year later. Ashton failed with Mephistopheles, who does not sufficiently command the action, but his lovers have a Romeo and Juliet quality of ill-starred, lyrical intensity and in the 1944 season they were beautifully played by Sally Gilmour and Robert Harrold, a youthful and undeveloped dancer with a *danseur noble* "line" and considerable technical possibilities.

Mephisto Valse, far more than any other ballet in the Rambert repertoire, quite definitely suggests the master choreographer who will prove capable of handling dancers *en masse* on a larger stage. I do not think this claim can be made in the same degree in respect of Andrée Howard; her guests in *Lady Into Fox* are not outstandingly well handled and in her more recent ballet, *Carnival of Animals*, produced at the Mercury Theatre in 1944, the general "messy" effect cannot be laid down entirely to the rather fussy costumes and over-crowded stage. As a children's entertainment this ballet has delightful touches—the Lion, the painfully lugubrious tortoises, the adorable Child of Sally Gilmour—but the playing of the Saint-Saëns music on a radiogram, never a satisfactory accompaniment to dance, mitigated against the effect of the production and the expressiveness of animal

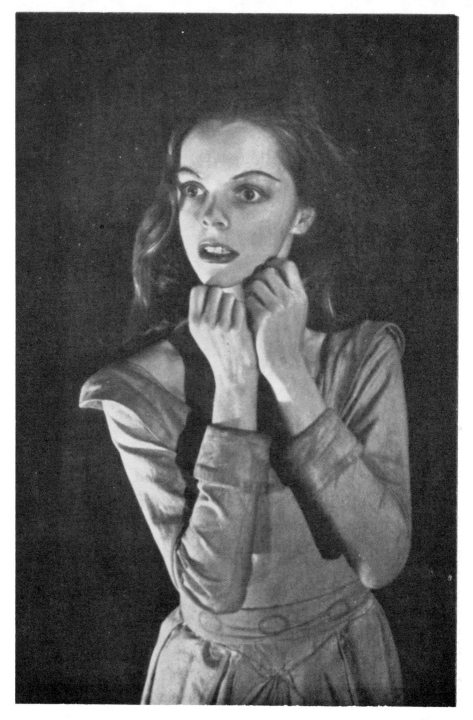

Confessional
Sally Gilmour

Plate LIV

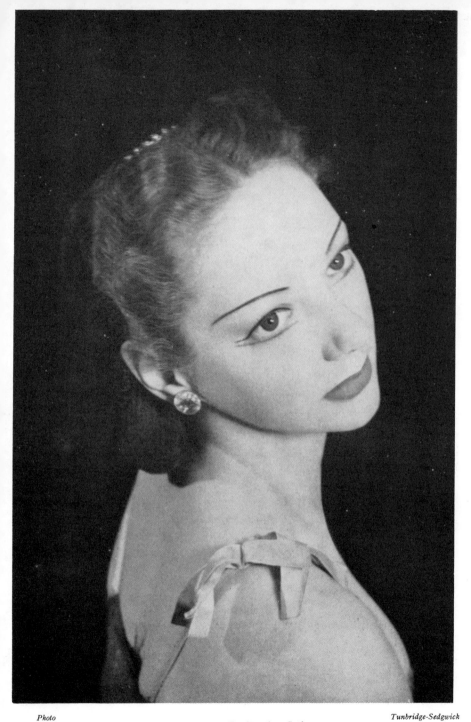

Jardin Aux Lilas
Joan McClelland as "The Woman in His Past"

Plate LV

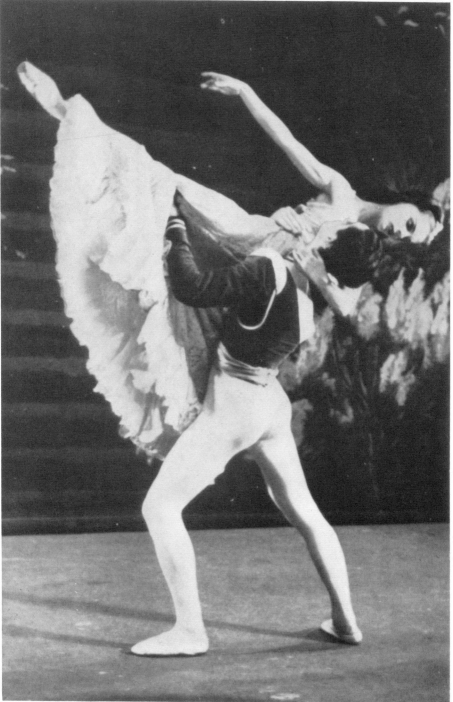

Jardin Aux Lilas
Sally Gilmour and Frank Staff

Plate LVI

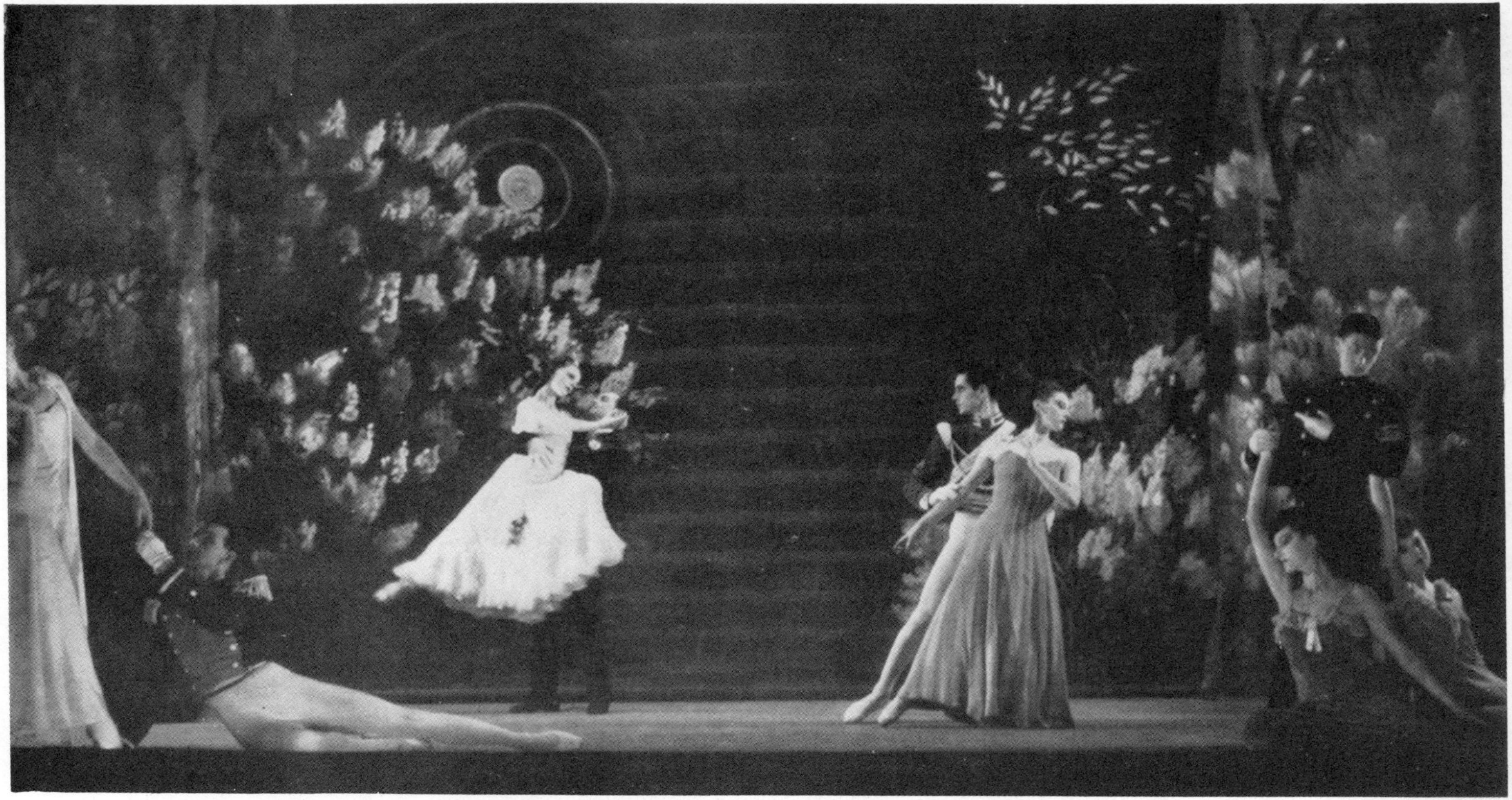

Photo *Tunbridge-Sedgwick*

Jardin Aux Lilas: Décor by Hugh Stevenson

Plate LVII

Action Photo
Peggy Delius

Plate LVIII

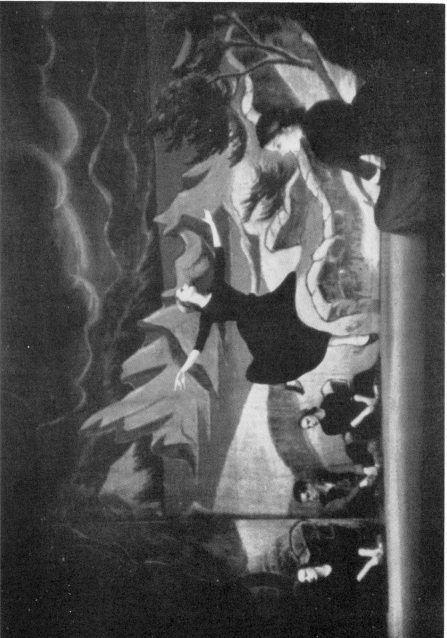

Dark Elegies
Sally Gilmour in
Variation.

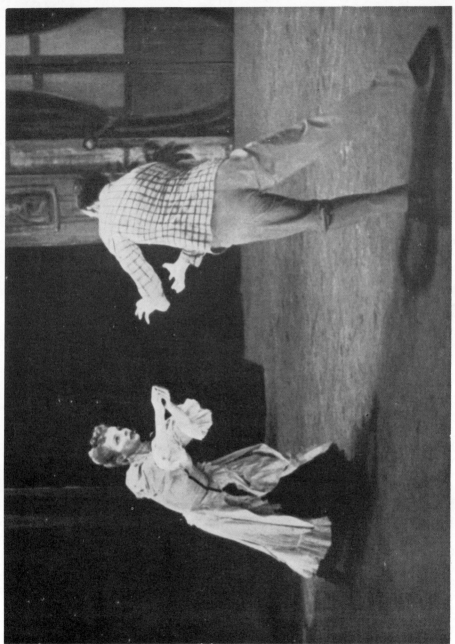

Lady Into Fox.
Transformation
scene: Sally
Gilmour and
Stanley Newby.

Plate LIX

Action Photo
G. B. L. Wilson

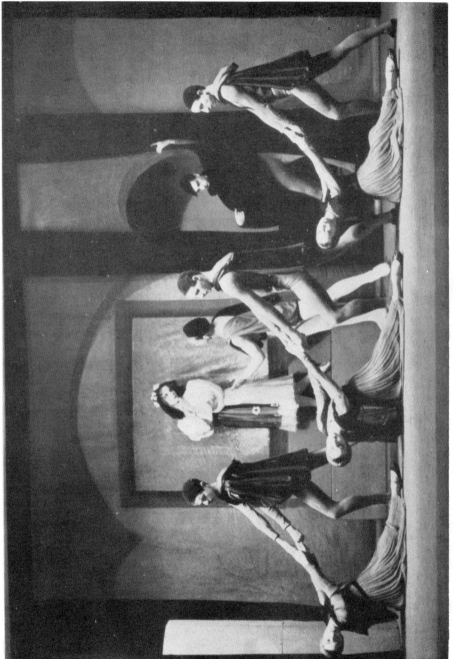

Mephisto Valse.
Arrangement of principals and *corps de ballet.*

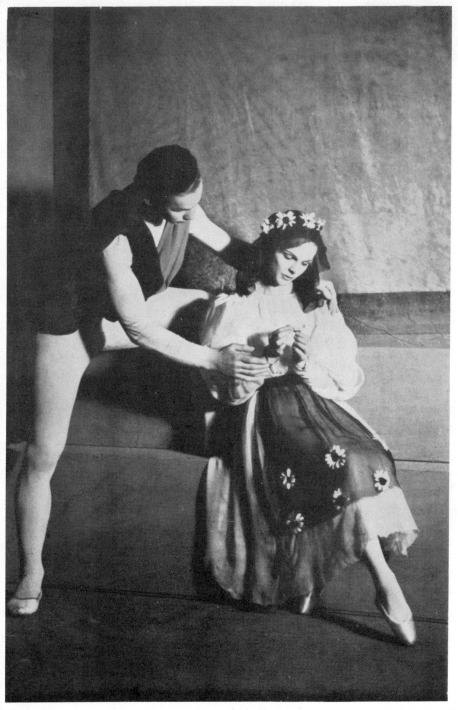

Photo

Tunbridge-Sedgwick

Mephisto Valse
Robert Harrold and Sally Gilmour

Plate LXI

movement in *Lady Into Fox*, or even the much earlier *Mermaid*, is not equalled here. The dances of the mermaids in this early ballet, performed in costumes which deliberately restrict the use of the legs, show real creative imagination in the suggestion of an atmosphere of restless undersea mobility; the dance flows sinuously through the entire body of the dancers, fingertips, arms and torso seeming to vibrate in the iridescent ocean-green light, and the mimed scene of the shipwreck, although requiring extreme care in performance to achieve its effect, contains some graphic invention. The chief defect of this Hans Andersen ballet is disjointedness: the narrative proceeds by jerks and in spite of the Mermaid's pathetic ineffectuality on dry land, and a varied *pas de deux* with her Prince, the final scene lacks dramatic climax and the characters never truly come to life.

Lady Into Fox, based on David Garnett's novel and the kind of fantasy that has always made particularly good subject matter for ballet, is much stronger dramatically, and the *pas de deux* work is notable, with some charming "lifts" and a linking of hands of husband and wife that anticipates Ashton in *The Quest*. The inexpressiveness of the dance of the Huntsman that precipitates the tragedy is unfortunate, but it is counterbalanced by the brilliantly-conceived movement for the Fox, an unusual piece of dance characterisation in which the change from feminine to vixenish ferocity is startlingly shown both by the choreographer and the dancer, Sally Gilmour. Robert Harrold's performance of the husband in this ballet was also eloquent and moving. Honneger's music, with its eerie atonality, was an admirable choice for such a fantasy and Andrée Howard's musical feeling is still more strikingly shown in *Death and the Maiden*, in which the spirit of Schubert's music, the *andante cantabile* from the Quartet in D Minor, is vividly captured in movement and theme. This ballet shows how remarkably, and with great simplicity of means, Tragedy may be condensed into a small framework without losing any of its potency. The elongated shadow of the figure of Death, the quick sunlit lyricism of the girl's first entrance, her fading strength and mad whirl to escape, the limp fall of her hand at the icy touch of Death, are imagined in dance with moving sensibility. The introduction of the classical arabesque into the otherwise supple movement of the black-cloaked *corps de ballet* is the only flaw in this ballet's consistency of style.

More fluid in progression than *Lady Into Fox*, *Death and the Maiden* is, both musically and emotionally, the most satisfying and complete of all Andrée Howard's ballets, although in her new work, *The*

Fugitive, based on a theme by Hugh Stevenson with music by Leonard Salzedo, she handles her *corps de ballet* of ball-dancers, in a magnificent slow rumba, with a finer sense of sustained atmosphere and complex movement than ever before. This drama of two sisters who hide a fugitive from justice, with all the consequent repercussions of love, fear, jealousy and betrayal, has excellent qualities of human interest and suspense; its chief defects are the insufficiently defined psychology of the elder sister, with her abrupt change of character under the influence of thwarted passion, and a lack of dramatic and plastic contrast between the dancing of the sisters and that of the wounded and exhausted fugitive, whose movement is as restless and energetic as theirs. The eloquent contrast of mobility and stillness that gives such expressiveness to Ashton's ballets, and which Miss Howard achieved through the figure of the husband in *Lady Into Fox*, is lacking here, and the first scene as a result becomes too feverish an exposition of dance for dancing's sake. It is a fairly common tendency in the choreography produced for this company and gives the work of the various choreographers, at times, a curious similarity of dance idiom. Marie Rambert's own passionate interest in classical technique, and the omission from her productions of *Swan Lake* of the mime passages, a basic experience in controlled and expressive gesture her artists have always lacked, may have had some influence in this. Hugh Stevenson's costumes and scenery for *The Fugitive*, deliberately indefinite in period, have an attractive warmth of colouring and the parts of the fugitive and two sisters were finely created by Walter Gore, Sally Gilmour and Joan McClelland. This ballet is not choreographically on the plane of Tudor's *Jardin Aux Lilas* and Ashton's still greater *Nocturne*, both of which it resembles in its setting of a ball during which a human drama is enacted, but it shows a new facet of Miss Howard's skill and a far stronger sense of drama and *corps de ballet* pattern than in her last few works.

Antony Tudor's *Dark Elegies*, ambitiously set to Mahler's *Kinder-totenlieder*, is a dance tragedy of sombre simplicity, and although its success is not complete it is a work showing flashes of power and beauty of movement. There is nothing new in the idealisation of the peasant by the intelligentsia; it is as old as Millet and the French Revolution. Tudor's peasants, heroic in bereavement and with a uniform intensity of facial expression, escape pretentiousness only by a thread, and his use of classical pointwork in solo and *pas de deux* conflicts in style with the folk dance ideology of the work as a whole.

The folk dance figurations are, however, used with originality and a stark force of reiteration, the music is often sensitively paralleled (one movement of the hand tracing an imaginary line and tangent is particularly memorable) and the basis of the dances in religious ritual is finely realised when one of the men, dervish-like, lashes the dancers into a rushing circle of excitement.

Jardin Aux Lilas is a less ambitious but more well-knit work in which Hugh Stevenson's *décor*, heavy with the bloom and almost with the scent of lilac, Chausson's music and Tudor's choreography are finely correlated. This tragedy of a marriage of convenience is movingly suggested by means of fleeting contacts and interruptions, the touching of hands, simple plastic lines and a rich and dramatic use of "lifts." It has something of the tragic irony of de Maupassant and the dramatic characterisation of Balzac, and Sally Gilmour as the Bride and Joan McClelland as the discarded mistress have in recent productions played with a poignant but sharply contrasted intensity. *Jardin Aux Lilas*, which has achieved success in America under the title of *Lilac Garden*, gives superb body to the Ballet Rambert programmes and its lyrical and bitter grief is movingly concentrated by Sally Gilmour into one sudden moment of desolate immobility.

A more recent revival of Tudor's *Descent of Hebe* has emphasised the extremely variable quality of this choreographer's work, partly owing to his slowness in finding his true style, that of psychological dance-drama. Ballet has long since outgrown its mythological period and it is surprising that this tedious legend, in which the characters have no psychological interest and in which the dance is over-full of classroom *clichés*, should have been created as late as 1935, only one year before the masterly *Jardin Aux Lilas* and actually a year later than *The Planets*, in which the movement and groupings are far more original, flexible and expressive. *Hebe*'s sole claim to interest to-day is in the striking *décor* for the Night sequence, though Nadia Benois's designs for the rest of the ballet are less attractive. *The Planets*, based on the music of Gustav Holst, is also helped by a truly magnificent *décor*, in which Hugh Stevenson has achieved a fine sense of limitless space. Though the "Mars" and "Mercury" scenes are not entirely successful—the first notably lacks the conflict implicit in the planet of War and the movement tends to be monotonous, unnatural and over-strained in its virility—the first, "Venus," has a lyrical feeling for the theme and the last, "Neptune," is better still, creating an undersea atmosphere with some fluent lines and movements of great beauty and musicality. The chief protagonist has been very finely danced by Joan McClelland, a dancer of exceptional control and dramatic range. Her *vignette* of a fading *cocotte* in *Judgment of Paris* shows a searching and bitterly ironic sense of tragedy and lifts this sordid little study of a Paris brothel to an artistic plane to which it does not rightfully belong.

I cannot look on this work, or on *Gala Performance*, as anything but retrograde steps in Tudor's career, though the second earns its place in the programme because of its fun of situation, intensified in recent performances by Sally Gilmour's sparkling impertinence and Joan McClelland's deadly unapproachability and poise as the ballerina from Milan. A burlesque of the coquettish inanities of Continental ballet during the last century, and of the rivalries of factious ballerinas, it is unbalanced by the choice of music, Prokofiev's "Classical Symphony" being a charming *pastiche* of Mozartian elegancies and totally unsuitable in character and period-style for such a theme. What was required was the tinkling vacuity of inferior Délibes. *Gala Performance* demands a high standard of technique in performance which in war-time it could not receive, but choreographically it is undistinguished, and a comparison between Tudor's difficult but boring classical *adagio* and Ashton's richly inventive and witty one in *The Wedding Bouquet* shows how little Tudor's talents lie in the direction of parody or classical *pas*. *Jardin Aux Lilas* would retain its quality on any stage or in any company, and in his American ballets, *Pillar of Fire* and *Dim Lustre*, Tudor appears to have reverted to his gift for psychological suggestion and drama. Tudor's choreography shows an occasional forcing or awkwardness of movement and lack of ease in transition between steps and groups. Both probably spring from a too early concentration on choreography at the expense of his work as a dancer, for a sound knowledge of the physical possibilities of movement is best based on extensive personal experience of dancing. But undoubtedly Tudor's is a brain to be reckoned with in modern ballet, although the determination of his admirers to read into his slightest work a rather alarming social significance threatens to make him, in England, a *coterie* figurehead rather than a choreographer of the wider popularity his gifts demand.

Frank Staff, who also had his first opportunities in this company, is a young choreographer still to some extent in the immature stage. He has wit in abundance, but seems to lack depth or true musicality as distinct from facility of rhythm. This musical lack is noticeable at some points in *Peter and the Wolf*, particularly in respect of the dances of the Wolf and the Bird where the orchestration seems to call for movement of greater complexity and invention. Otherwise this is a merry and charming charade for children of which the outstanding features are the delightful Prokofiev music and commentary, the enchantingly drawn Peter (Sally Gilmour is a completely convincing little Russian tow-haired boy), and the comic Hunters, led by Frank Staff himself with a dazzling absurdity. Guy Sheppard's expressionistic *décor* gives the ballet exactly the right simplicity.

The chief charm of Staff's other principal ballet, *Czernyana*, is its infectious high spirits. It is gay and sly dance parody, flagging once or twice into classroom tediousness but at its best first-rate, with a delicious choice of prancing music and a skit of the Symphonic Ballet that has a riotous mock-intensity. Staff dances the *Se Habla Espanol* with a wicked Ashton-pointed malice, Sally Gilmour has a moment or two of inane insouciance, and Elizabeth's Schooling's classical burlesque is a brilliantly-timed piece of sheer silliness. This last dancer has a mischievous sense of fun which is also at its best in Staff's little Scottish *divertissement, The Tartans,* and as the débutante in *Façade,* although her performances in Ninette de Valois's *Bar Aux Folies-Bergère* and in *Death and the Maiden* show her to have a wider range.

In a more recent ballet, *Un Songe,* produced in 1945, Staff has followed the tradition of Balanchine's *Cotillon*. A dance study designed to create a mood or atmosphere rather than a theme, it had great imagination in the opening dream sequence, danced without music to emphasise the uncanny and macabre effect, but its lack of any dramatic contrast or climax, and the ineffectuality of its characters, caused it to peter out without significance. It was, however, beautifully produced and lit and showed something of Staff's talent and possibilities.

Walter Gore's *Confessional,* produced in 1941, has a deeper emotional content than anything yet produced by Staff. It is a tragic monologue of ballet, mimed to music by Sibelius and a bitter poem by Robert Browning, a narration of past events which hammer in the rebellious and distracted mind of a young girl imprisoned by religious bigotry. The tragic impact of the poem and Sally Gilmour's superb delineation of wasting pain, dead passion and delirium give this work a power which is almost completely independent of the choreography. The ballet is little more than a mime creation for one character, with a fleeting tender interlude when the girl remembers her dead lover and

re-enacts in her dream a tragic episode in their story; but within its
limits the movement is sensitively reflective of the mood and rhythm of
poem and music and in its construction the work is entirely original.

Gore's first ballet after his release from the Royal Navy proved a
much lighter work. *Simple Symphony*, a nautical dance suite composed
to Benjamin Britten's music, echoes the simplicity of the title and
the light, rhythmic charm of the music in an arrangement of dances
notable for their good humour, consistency of style and continuity
of progression. The "sentimental saraband," in which these joyous
and impudent fisherfolk take on a *Dark Elegies* gravity, more Tudor
than Trafalgar, is the least original movement. The rest has the
salty freshness of a sea breeze and a variety in rustic dance movement
that is enhanced in charm by the *décor* and costumes of the young
designer Ronald Wilson.

In its classical and Fokine revivals this company is inevitably
limited by the size of the stages on which it often performs as well as
the lack of a good orchestra and the inexperience of the company in
such work. *Les Sylphides*, as performed by this company, is notably
musical and has the right feeling in mood and decoration; what is
lacking is that delicate poetic ethereality which can only be attained
when the dancers, in physique as well as style, are essentially suited
to romantic dancing of the Taglioni tradition. Only Sally Gilmour
has shown this quality in war-time performances, and her feathery
grace is wholly exquisite. The dancing of the *corps de ballet* in *Swan
Lake* has also shown a pattern and breadth of style that are a credit to
Madame Rambert's teaching, although here again the solo work is
less good, Sally Gilmour making her début as the Swan Princess with
an unexpected sense of the classical spirit in carriage and sweep of
arm but necessarily lacking speed and polish of technique. Small and
compactly built, with beautifully arched insteps, she is a dancer of
considerable charm, but it is as a character-mime that she principally
shines. In dramatic expression, although not in dancing powers, she
takes her place beside Margot Fonteyn. Only her petal-like grace,
and Joan McClelland's placid and beautifully-controlled dancing as
Chiarina, saved this company's *Carnaval* from complete disaster.
The company lacks not only the resources but also the professional
finish in presentation for such a work; character make-up is markedly
poor, greybeards with faces as fresh as a May morning being the rule,
and although double piano work well executed is infinitely preferable
to a poor orchestra, there is no doubt the lack of instrumentation

gave a certain feeling of thinness to the choreography. It is not by accident that *Jardin Aux Lilas*, in which the music was scored for violin as well as piano, gave an impression of richness and drama in the dance that was until recently lacking in the production of most of the other ballets. These are weaknesses that must be faced, however strong a company may be in essentials.

These essentials are good dancing standards and, above all, a high level of original choreography. This company possesses the first, even though it may not at the moment possess the dancers to enforce them, and it maintains the second through a repertoire of unusual variety and extensiveness, one which provides an interesting chronological *résumé* of English choreography although since the greatest ballets of Frederick Ashton and Ninette de Valois, composed for another company, and the ballets of Robert Helpmann cannot be included the *résumé* is necessarily incomplete. A number of ballets in the Ballet Rambert repertoire are immature works created before the choreographer had attained full powers of expression or dramatic cohesion; they are historically revealing and interesting for this reason. The ballets which are complete artistic entities and unmistakably adult are fewer in number, but it is they that hold the repertoire firmly together and justify Marie Rambert's policy of giving the young choreographer the means to test and develop his creative ability.

Service to an art is not merely a matter of concrete achievement but of *paving the way* for such achievement. This is the service that Marie Rambert has rendered in such an extensive degree to English ballet: she has not merely made the considerable achievements of her own company possible, she has been frequently instrumental in making possible the achievements of others. It is her tragedy that with her passion for and understanding of the classical ballet she has never had the resources to enable her to stage such ballets on an adequate scale; but in a sense her loss has been Ballet's gain, for she has been forced to concentrate her whole tremendous enthusiasm and flair for inspiring talent on the building up of fresh choreography and the development of the quite new and subtle style-form of chamber ballet. Her influence in this has been the more valuable because she is able to temper her enthusiasm and encouragement with criticism: no ballet of an immature choreographer reaches her stage unless the rehearsals satisfy her that the work is of sufficient quality to warrant inclusion in the repertoire. Although this process of selection and rejection may, probably, mean that a choreographer sometimes feels his venturesomeness is being cramped, it has ensured that no work in the Ballet Rambert repertoire falls below a certain standard of competence. There are fewer ballet companies of which one can say this than one would think.

The Ballet Rambert now aims at expansion; if it is to continue to perform the classics a full orchestra and a stronger company of good dancers are indeed essential, and dancers are not easily attracted into a company which has not the resources to give them major opportunities and to secure "dates" in leading theatres. The artistic security of this company up to now has rested in the fact that generally speaking it has not challenged comparison with a major company such as Sadler's Wells but has developed a line of its own in the production of *ballet intime* and the encouragement of young choreographers. This is a side of the company's work it would be a misfortune, both to English ballet as a whole and to the company itself, to abandon; there is a need in England for an experimental theatre providing opportunities for the young artist of ballet to learn his job. As long as this policy is retained the Ballet Rambert will still hold a place in English ballet in its own right and not become just a rather unnecessary twin of the full-scale National ballet developed by Ninette de Valois at Sadler's Wells.

CHAPTER XVII

BALLETS JOOSS

THE Ballets Jooss is the only foreign ballet company that has been seen in England during the war years, and although it falls outside the classical ballet tradition its importance in the history of twentieth-century choreography is considerable enough to make its inclusion essential in any serious study of ballet in England to-day. After a prolonged tour of North and South America early in the war the company made its London reappearance at the Haymarket Theatre in the summer of 1944. The last London season of the Ballets Jooss had been in 1939, and therefore this application of the Central European non-classical dance technique to ballet form was a new experience for a large proportion of the present-day ballet audience.

Founded and held together by the creative power of one man, Kurt Jooss, the Ballets Jooss had its beginnings in Essen twenty years ago, and its first international success with its production of *The Green Table* in 1932, when this ballet secured first prize in the International Congress of the Dance in Paris. Jooss, a pupil of the Hungarian Rudolph Laban, whose discoveries in movement and physique he developed and evolved into a comprehensive system of dance training and technique, has aimed at the creation of a form of dance more natural to contemporary life than the artificial restrictions of classical ballet as he understands it, and although he has taken many movements and positions from classical technique he has discarded the blocked shoe, obvious solo work and purity of "line" in its classic sense. Suppleness, control and extreme lightness (aided by the use of a carpet on the stage, which would be an impossibility in the speedier and more intricate execution of classical *pas*) are the salient features of Jooss-trained dancers, together with a teamwork that ensures the balance of the ballet as a whole. The aim in the choreography has been an extension of the demand for dramatic expression made by the great reformers of classical ballet, Noverre and Fokine, the complete elimination of virtuosity, the merging of mime and dance, and the maintenance of a continuity of movement entirely free from the sustained poses and preparations of classical ballet. To a large extent Jooss, by his own genius in the creation of a balletic theme, as well as by his Hogarthian sense that "the line of beauty is a curve," has succeeded in creating a contemporary ballet movement of vitality and expressiveness and an ensemble of dancers of unusual artistry and precision; his failure is in his lack of appreciation of the fact that the classical ballet, through its best choreographers, has equally been able to achieve artistic progression, drama and fluidity of movement, and to absorb from all schools of dance, while retaining its full materials for the creation of contrast, variety and brilliance when these may be demanded by the nature of the ballet or the theme. It is this contrast of brilliance that Jooss, in his reaction against the empty virtuosity of classicism as he first saw it (probably not under its best and most progressive conditions) has deliberately sacrificed; his contrast is largely of the beautiful and the grotesque, upturned toes and angular movements being freely used in his ballets to suggest contrasts of character and strength, very notably in the part of Death in *The Green Table* and in the dances of the peasants in *The Seven Heroes*.

It is curious that so astute a mind, having recognised the dramatic necessity for contrasts of movement in the depiction of character, should have failed to recognise the necessity for contrasts of *speed* in the creation of atmosphere. The rounded and unhurried grace of the Jooss school of movement needs the balance of strong clean lines and swiftness of action to stress its beauty, just as feminine dancing needs the balance of masculine strength to enhance its special qualities and achieve a richer orchestration of dance movement. Clarity and virility of line is occasionally achieved, notably in the dances of the Standard Bearer and soldiers in *The Green Table*, but swiftness and brilliance of turn and beat are not possible under Jooss's self-imposed limitations of technique. Prince Serge Wolkonsky, in his manifesto on the Ballets Jooss, wrote that they had "introduced into choreography that which was lacking in the classical ballet; truthfulness to life; absence of insipid affectation; mimicry based upon the laws of nature." But ballet, whatever form it may take, is by its very nature a theatrical convention, and unless it can be accepted that human beings express themselves through dance and movement and never through speech its truthfulness to life can only be relative. Of what, then, does this *relative* truthfulness to life consist? What are, from the balletic point of view, "the laws of nature"? Surely an *impression* of human life, a heightened reality, and certain impressions of life the Ballets Jooss have achieved with vividness and poignancy. But nature has also violence, exhilaration, excitement, passion and sparkle, and these are qualities which tend to become so intellectualised in Jooss' ballets that they lose their potency. The fault is probably as much that of the choreographer as of the system, for no one choreographer is likely to be equally facile in the expression of all of the human passions and aspects of life; but in view of the claims made it is imperative that it should be pointed out, in fairness to those classical choreographers who have also created successful impressions of life and human character, with the greater variety of movement at their disposal.

Classical companies can perhaps learn most from the Ballets Jooss in the question of musical rhythm; this Jooss, through his dancers, has brought to a degree of accuracy and subtlety unmatched in classical companies as a whole, and the hesitant poses of Death in *The Green Table* solo, the negation of Jooss's general view that movement should be continuous, are a direct acknowledgment that the laws of music and character may override dance theory. To the laws of linear beauty Jooss will not make such concessions and when he takes a classical ballet pose, the arabesque, and through the figure of Psyche in *Pandora* attempts to merge it into the motion of her dance, the quality of the pose becomes blurred and its loveliness lost. From the point of view of visual taste Jooss's selection of classical steps to be included in his work is curiously variable; he has retained from classical ballet some of its less attractive technicalities—the awkward *pliés à la seconde*, outturned feet and fifth positions which are relegated as far as possible to the classroom by the more advanced of classical choreographers—and it is these that seem to me to create flaws in the fluid dance structure composed with such sensitivity at times by Jooss from his own repertoire of movement. He has at once taken too much from classical ballet and too little. His greatest contribution to ballet is not visual, although he has composed many moving pictures and much dancing of charm and emotional expression; it is in his recognition of dance as a vital medium for the depiction of contemporary life and character, and of ballet as a coherent art which may only evolve from the close collaboration of musician, designer, choreographer and stage technician.

The Ballets Jooss, relying not on scenery but on lighting to convey the atmosphere of the theme, have brought to a fine art the use of a spotlight and graded colouring to accentuate the important figures in a group and to combine dramatic with pictorial effect. The costumes are designed simultaneously with, or after, the creation of the choreography, and with a full knowledge on the part of the designer of the movement and grouping they must enhance and reveal. The music, where possible, is similarly composed in collaboration with the choreographer, though there is a danger-signal here of too complete a domination of the choreographer at the expense of the musician's creative imagination. The standard of the music, judged by concert values, created for the Ballets Jooss is not high and the relationship of choreographer and composer in this company seems nearer to that of Petipa and Tchaikovsky than that of Fokine and Stravinsky. The ideal Jooss score remains that of F. A. Cohen for *The Green Table*, where the music has rhythmic and dramatic values that the choreographer is particularly well equipped to reflect in movement.

The Green Table remains Jooss's greatest and most powerful work, a satire which suggests the vicious recurring circle of peace conference and war with virulent irony, and in a series of poignant groupings and dances pictures the futile tragedy and horror of war. Symbolic and expressionistic in style, it yet shirks no reality to which the passions of war give rise, from the rapacity of the profiteer and deadly contagion of the brothel to the suffering of the women and martyrdom of the guerrilla. The choreography of this ballet is more robust, more vivid in its delineation of evil, than in any of Jooss's later works, and in the masterly first and last scenes of the "Gentlemen in Black," a satiric comment on the mailed fist beneath the velvet glove in diplomatic green table discussions, the concentration on masked head, hands and arms is used to build up a graphic suggestion of eloquence and dissension. The living and prophetic impact of this ballet is, if anything, heightened by present conditions and the grief of the women and Death's leading of his victims, in a single macabre line, across the stage remain among the most moving scenes in modern ballet. Jooss's own creation of Death, a juggernaut of the machine age, has a robot-like force and it is the measure of his imagination that he is able to show Death not only as a symbol of Mars, the terrible God of War, but also as the giver of peace. Death's lifting of the Old Mother into his arms is, in this sense, a touch of sensitive insight.

The Big City, with its first scene in which the cross-currents of town life in the twenties are pictured with brilliant stylisation, is also one of the best of the earlier Jooss ballets. It is slick and facile as an American movie, and the merging kaleidoscope of the smart night club and apache haunt, the uncouth isolated pain of the deserted youth and the fleeting lyrical touch of his first encounter with the girl are finely touched in. The scene of the children has a perfectly-chiselled simplicity and the suspicious and protective working-class mothers are drawn with a witty but sympathetic observation. Jooss has never produced anything more gravely touching than this little stylised cameo of a scene. The ending of the ballet is a trifle indeterminate and depends entirely for its psychological clarity on the expression in the face of the Young Girl before she rushes disillusioned from the futile physical excesses of the night club. Noëlle de Mosa, a dancer of grace and sensibility, has played this part exquisitely, and Hans Zullig makes the Young Workman the key figure of the ballet, inarticulate yet deeply expressive. His little shiver as of cold, at the end, is a touch of delicate imagination.

The Prodigal Son is also a major ballet with a dramatically expressive opening and ending which show the Prodigal's departure from and return to his parents. Jooss's hand movements as the Father are exquisitely stylised and the Mother's cradling of an imaginary baby in the last scene is a characteristic Jooss touch. The son's change of character, with the acquisition of power, is not psychologically well explained and a Mysterious Stranger is confusingly introduced, although this part excitingly exploits Hans Zullig's magnificent control and technique; but the revolutionary scenes are planned with a greater intricacy of mass movement than in any of Jooss' other ballets and the flux and flow of the mob are vividly maintained.

Of Jooss's less serious ballets *A Spring Tale* suffers, like much of his work, from excessive length and repetition; a charming fairy story, it is of too frail a texture to withstand such prolonged treatment and the wood scenes need a more varied and imaginative choreography to hold both eye and interest. The ceremonial of a Court of women is satirised with a brilliant *grotesquerie;* Jooss's sense of fun here is unbounded and his shy little princess, in her cap like the calyx of a flower, is an amused and tender creation to which Ulla Soederbaum has given, in some enchanting performances, a harebell charm. Hans Zullig displays as her Prince that fairy-tale chivalry and elegance that in classical ballet are the true prerogative of the *danseur noble;* this superb dancer has line and style in everything he touches. It is just because they have been produced with the dramatic brevity *A Spring Tale* lacks that *Ballade* and *Pavane*, less charming but more coherent and artistically balanced works, grapple the interest without slackening throughout the performance. *Ballade*, the story of a Queen who murders her young and reluctant rival for the King's affection with the gift of a poisoned bouquet, is a wordless drama of strong characterisation and magnificently sustained tension. There is no entrance in ballet handled more dramatically than that of the Queen in *Ballade*, menace in every line from the proud tilted head to the inturned wrists. Played in recent performances by Maria Fedro and Kurt Jooss, both the Queen and King have a sharp-cut arrogance that slashes like a sword through the lyrical passages between the Marquis and his bride. The contrast of mood packed into this tiny work is astonishing, for it is maintained in spite of a musical score of such a cacophonous lack of variety that only a mind such as that of Jooss, who feels that the function of the choreographer is not to express the music but merely to parallel its rhythm, could probably have overridden it and preserved the dramatic balance of his story. A certain monotony of leg movement, derived from a concentration on a form of *battement*, is a choreographic flaw which passes practically unnoticed in the finely planned construction of the action, and in the figure of the Marquis here, as in that of the Young Workman in *Big City*, Jooss has displayed that essence of good choreography whether the technique be classical or free dance, the ability to make one motionless character an expressive centrifugal point of the surrounding action. The helpless acquiescence and grief of the young Marquis are conveyed in a taut line of body and pose, and his turn towards the King and Queen in the final tableau, with the body of his dead bride at his feet, is a mute accusation. The part is beautifully played by Zullig, who points the tragedy with the restraint and economy of gesture that inform all his work.

Pavane, a twin work to *Ballade* in scale and style, has the same dramatic economy; it is the most satisfying musically of all Jooss's works and movingly parallels Ravel in its picture of the young Infanta crushed beneath the inhuman formality of the Spanish Court. The part makes demands of pathos on the actress that have not been met in recent performances, but here as in *Ballade* the staging of the Court is given a decorative shimmer by the simple but effective use of cellulose in the costume design. With Jooss cheapness never becomes obvious or causes a deterioration to the vulgar or the drab; as a stage director he has a constant freshness of invention, and if only his company accepted the formula that *décor*, as well as costume design, is an integral part of balletic unity his supervision would doubtless ensure some stage pictures of still greater atmosphere and power. As it is the use of curtains as a background makes, in the long run, for a certain one-dimensional effect which is not essentially the fault of the choreography, although when a hint of stylised scenery is added, as in the nautical symbols of Sigurd Leeder's *Sailor's Fancy* and in the charming wrought-iron park gate of Hans Zullig's *Le Bosquet*, the impression can be one of wit or charm.

The rather crude dining table and tree introduced into Jooss's recent *Company at the Manor* are less successful, although Doris Zinkeison's costumes charmingly capture the Dickensian note of the theme Jooss has superimposed, not always happily, on to Beethoven's "Spring" Sonata in F Major. This work of the youthful Beethoven has a vernal lightness of touch that cannot be fitted to such literal fancies as Victorian coquettries, comic butlers and matchmaking papas and mamas, and Jooss's introduction of a flamboyant Brazilian suitor to one of the most lyrical passages of the music is a musical lapse over which even Zullig, Massine-like in impudence, cannot skate without an audible cracking of ice. The dream-like *andante* and the galloping coach drive are nearer the spirit of the music, and divorced from its score this would be a delightful light ballet with some choreography, including a cleverly-mimed coach drive, of genuine wit. Zullig dances with meticulously-timed comedy and precision and Noëlle de Mosa displays as always a limpid softness of movement. The ballet shows an increase in sparkle as compared with the earlier *Ball in Old Vienna*, although in audacity of invention *The Seven Heroes*, revived since the Haymarket season, remains incomparable among the Jooss comedies. The accent on grotesque movement is completely appropriate to the characterisation of Grimm's valorous-intentioned peasants and their wives; the style of the dance fits the ballet like a glove and the choreography has a facile variety that is both humorous and unforced. Yet here again the choice of music pulls the entire ballet out of shape, for the courtly English elegance of Purcell's music belongs in spirit to a class and period remote from this world of Central European peasants.

The technical progression of the Jooss system of dance, which seemed for some years to have become clogged and static, is also apparent in the only serious ballet Jooss produced during the war, *Pandora*. The use of dancers in the mass here shows an increased feeling for line and flexibility of composition, with a contrapuntal suggestion, lacking before, which may be the unconscious result of the inclusion of percussion in the score. The Hindu influence in the hand movements of Pandora, with the upturned palm that in the dances of antiquity and the Orient represents the vanity of the woman with a looking glass, is interesting as an indication of the way in which dance origins may penetrate into the newest choreographic forms, and there is one moment of superb imagination when Pandora, the evil genius of the world, sits on the monsters she has let loose and breathes with them in a mighty and terrifying undulation. Yet the ballet fails because its interest is purely that of abstract movement; its aim as a great dramatic allegory is vitiated in a series of long-drawn-out episodes in which the climax is so long delayed that it misfires when it comes. The characters are symbolic, reiterative and lacking in force, a great deal of the movement is meaningless and the passion of the bacchanal and the miseries of earthly evil are presented with an intellectualised stylisation that defeats its dramatic object. Jooss has nothing new to add to what he has already said in *The Green Table* about the bereavement of women in war; the part played by women in his ballets, unless it is one of seduction, is almost invariably passive and it is the man who displays character and acts as an individual.[1] The paucity and repetition of the choreography prevent the figures of the Youth and Psyche, the regenerative force in mankind, from acquiring any active spiritual value, and the effect of the ballet as a whole is one of emotional aridity, *The Green Table* without the guts. It is disappointing to have to write this because there is no doubt of the ambitious nature of the work, and its beauty at times as a spectacle (the lighting, the masks of Hein Heckroth and the seductive splash of colour in the costume of Pandora are masterly). The time, perhaps, is past when a comment on human ethics can have any force if wrapped up in the obscurities of Greek mythological allegory. If Jooss can combine his increasing freedom of technique with more of the dramatic pungency of *The Green Table*, and harness his fatal propensity to repetition, he may yet produce his masterpiece and justify his school as a progressive movement outside the classical tradition.

There is no doubt something of this lack of progression up to now (for *The Green Table*, produced in 1932, is still the best ballet in the repertoire) has been due to the fact that the movement has been forced

[1] This Germanic outlook of Jooss on women was immediately pointed out by an alert body of A.T.S. at a lecture on ballet, with the rider that when the woman's place was not obviously in the home, to mourn or be domesticated, she was usually a woman of the streets: "and German prostitutes are never successful"!

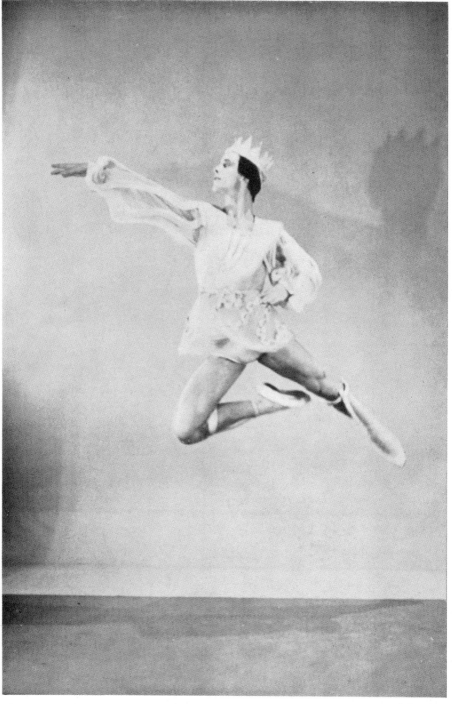

A Spring Tale
Hans Zullig as the Prince

Plate LXII

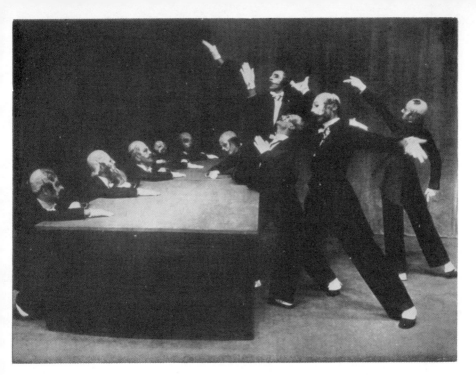

The Green Table

Plate LXIII   (*Above*) The Gentlemen in Black
Plate LXIV   (*Below*) March of the Dead: Kurt Jooss as Death

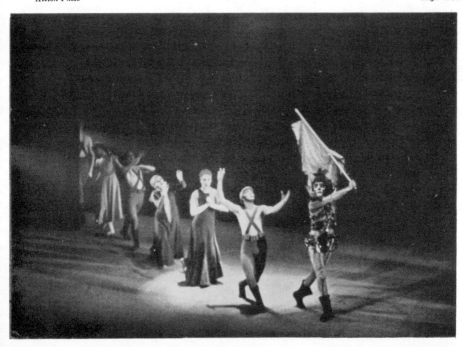

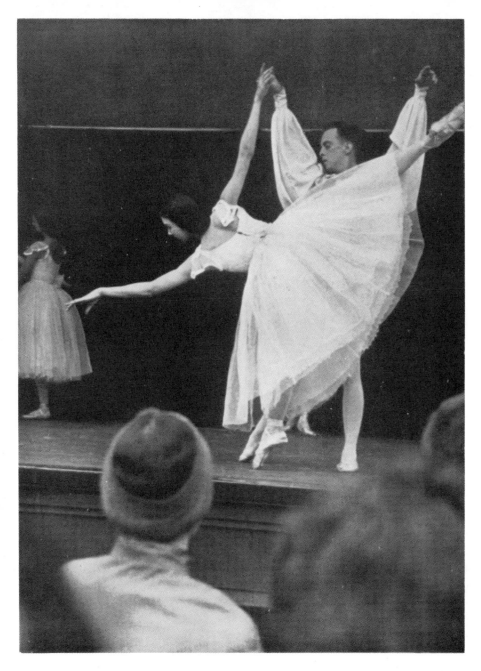

Les Sylphides at Victoria Park
Beryl Grey and Robert Helpmann

Plate LXV

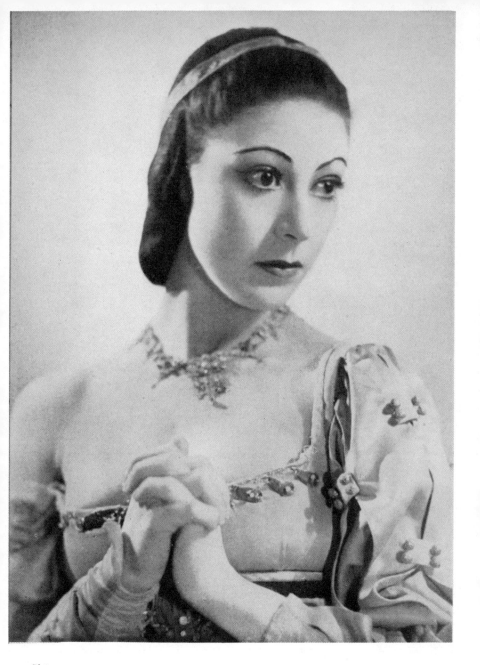

Head of a Dancer
Margot Fonteyn in *Hamlet*

Plate LXVI

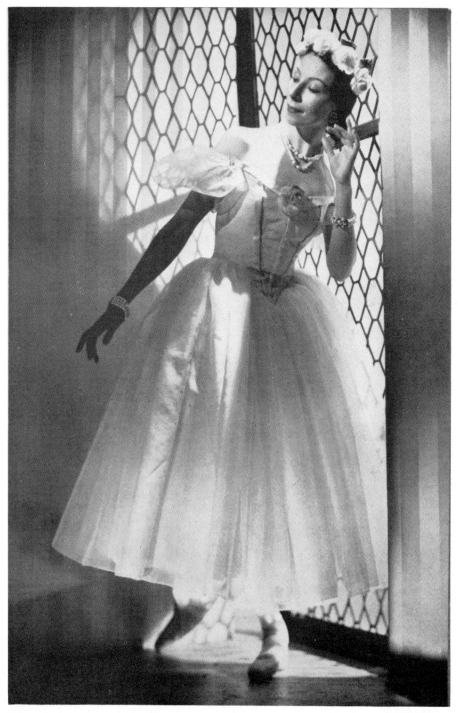

Photo

Ballet Theatre of New York
Alicia Markova in *Pas de Quatre*.

John E. Read

Plate LXVII

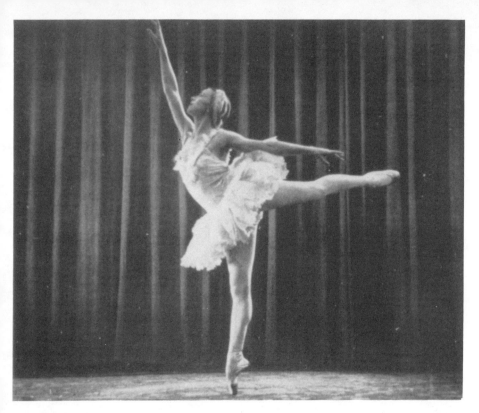

Plate LXVIII	(*Above*) Soviet Ballerina: Galina Ulanova in *Lac des Cygnes*
Plate LXIX	(*Below*) Dancers at Practice: Celia Franca and Anne Lascelles
Action Photo	*G. B. L. Wilson*

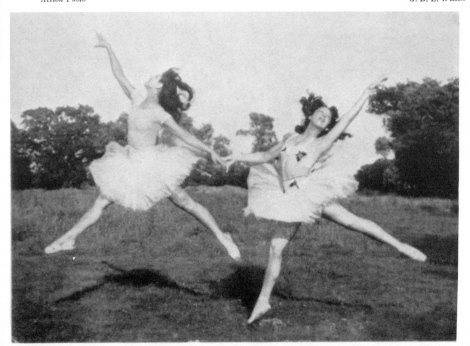

to rely on the work of one choreographer. No choreographic style, including the classical, could develop its full richness and variety under such circumstances, as new mentalities bring into every movement in art new directions and forms of expression. This Jooss himself fully realises, and the Ballets Jooss is on the threshold of an expansion which includes the encouragement of new choreographers from within its ranks. Sigurd Leeder's *Sailor's Fancy*, the first effort in this direction, was too near revue in style to suggest an influence of any importance, but Hans Zullig's first ballet, *Le Bosquet*, as slight in scale as all immature efforts should be, shows a freshness of attack and command of the Jooss dance material that strike a note of real hope for the future. None of the dancers, except Zullig himself, can quite capture the stylish elegancies of the Watteau scene; the Court dances of this period had already reached a degree of refinement that is more within the orbit of classical technique than the less formalised choreographic style of the Ballets Jooss. But Zullig has a painterly feeling for composition, and shows real talent in the maintenance of fluidity of movement from group to group. He tells his tale, the slight theme of a young girl who dreams of a past lover and awakes with a pang of disillusion and revulsion from her present admirer, with delicacy and point; the subject is suggested, rather than underlined, a useful gift in a choreographer, and the ending neatly sums up the theme. Doris Zinkeison's designs, after Watteau, add to the charm of the little work and although there is no sign, at present, of the Ballets Jooss producing a thinker of the capacity of Jooss himself—for there is no doubt of the brain behind the Jooss ballets—Zullig's ballet is an indication that the Jooss dance technique is flexible to a new approach; although like Jooss himself he produces his pictures mainly on the flat with little in the way of "lifts" or architecture of grouping. Zullig's greater interest in classical technique may, however, bring more of the rich accumulation of the past into this comparatively young technique, and Jooss himself, who like all reformers was obliged to break more violently with the past than his successors may need to do, recognises the possibility of this and has the breadth of mind to accede to it within reason.

For many years the world tours of this company made the possession of a full orchestra impossible; this has now been added and Jooss realises that the sustained melodic line of the stringed instruments will more clearly parallel the flowing continuity he aims at in his dance than the percussive qualities of the piano were able to do. As a choreographer he denies that choreography composed to an orchestral score may show the influence of the instrumentation in a richer counterpoint of movement than that composed to a piano score; but certainly all choreographers have not the same musical reactions in composition and the addition of an orchestra may influence the Jooss technique through other choreographers if not through Jooss himself.

The chief danger to this form of ballet is that of self-imposed obscurity; its admirers' total inability to admit any form of criticism of it whatsoever, and the tendency of all writing on the subject to smother it in "isms" and make a virtue of the fact that it is *"caviare to the general,"* are in reality very bad propaganda for the company's work and tend to alienate intelligent sections of the public to which the best of Jooss' ballets, if left to speak for themselves, would appeal. A ballet which can only be explained through complicated theorising on paper is a bad ballet, and it is the virtue of Jooss's best works that they have a simplicity and directness of emotional statement that represent an ideal fusion of thought and expression through movement. There is room for this form of ballet in the theatre even if one cannot accede that classical ballet is not equally able to treat of modern life and psychology within its own framework. *The Green Table* and *The Big City* have real contemporary relevance and it is to be hoped that the introduction of new choreographers will mean a renewal of such themes for ballet, for since these early productions this company has produced surprisingly little to justify its title of "the Contemporary Dance Theatre," and modern life is reflected in its later works only through the allegorical setting of another period.

BALLET AND THE FUTURE

CHAPTER XVIII

BALLET AND CONTEMPORARY LIFE

BALLET to-day is in many ways the most artistically vital branch of the theatre. The spoken drama produced little new work of any serious significance during the war, and until the Old Vic and John Gielgud seasons at the New and Haymarket theatres in 1944 the plays of Shakespeare and the great dramatists of the past were only rarely revived with any adequacy. Opera in this country has never produced any national school of composition and its repertoire in war-time shrunk to half a dozen of the more obvious foreign classics. Ballet alone has continued to produce new works by its best living creators, has kept its classics permanently in the repertoire and has drawn into the theatre first-class contemporary artists in other spheres.

Yet ballet, even more than the drama, has remained primarily escapist in its appeal, and though it occasionally touches the fundamentals of the human spirit it has rarely attempted any reflection of the problems and spiritual conflicts of our own time. *The Green Table*, with its scathing satire of the futility both of war and of Versailles, blazed a trail no choreographer, including its own, attempted seriously to follow until the production of *Miracle in the Gorbals* by the Sadler's Wells Company in 1944. Modern life, such as it is, has otherwise been mirrored only in its more chic, sophisticated and purely superficial aspects: wittily in *Façade*, with an erotic undercurrent in Nijinska's *The House Party*, but always touching only the smart fringe of humanity and the cheaper values and habits of the age. It is the *spirit* of the age, its search for a creed, the suffering of its war-ravaged peoples, its fight for freedom of mind and body, that has evaded the choreographer.

In six years of war and its aftermath only two ballets, *Dante Sonata* and *Adam Zero*, have even alluded to this major disaster which has affected the entire course of human existence. The Ballets Jooss, which might have been expected to record it, have produced a nautical farce, a Victorian comedy, a Watteau romance and one serious production, *Pandora*, in which the allusion to war is too tenebrous, brief and generalised to have an immediate significance. The Sadler's Wells Ballet have produced several works of major dramatic value, and in *The Prospect Before Us* at least Ninette de Valois has retained intact her facility as a translator of and commentator on English life and English art of another period. The English ballet's general concentration in fact has still been on the expression of the national spirit in literature and art *of the past*, and the message of England's greatness in Spenser's allegory of *The Faerie Queene*, as adapted by Ashton in *The Quest*, could touch us in war only at second remove. There is nothing against this reflection in ballet of our literary and artistic heritage; on the contrary it has given to English choreography a vital national style of its own. There is room, though, for the mirror to be held up to our own century as well as to those of the past, and it is because *Miracle in the Gorbals, Adam Zero* and *Dante Sonata* seem so unmistakably tragedies of our own time that they move many of us, in these days, more deeply than any other ballets, and give to the Sadler's Wells Ballet a link with human life not possessed by any other English company.

Miracle in the Gorbals is an example of how the realistic approach in setting and characterisation, heightened and theatricalised through the choreographic architecture and movement, may drive home the point of a modern morality as powerfully as the same approach in Hogarth's paintings and Ninette de Valois' ballet drove home the eighteenth-century morality of *The Rake's Progress*. This is the prose approach in ballet, equivalent to Ibsen in the drama and Tolstoy in literature; but in ballet as in drama and literature there is also the poetic approach, and it is perhaps its more poetic and deliberately abstract form of expression that gives to *Dante Sonata* its unchanging spiritual power. Its conflict of good and evil, the one continually tainted and submerged by the other and yet always breaking free and reaching towards a higher spiritual consciousness, is at once of our time and timeless. Its protagonists are symbols of human shame, suffering and malevolence which belong not merely to the clashing ideologies of the present day but to all such clashes of humanity down the ages; but they touch us the more nearly because we can also see in them individuals racked by our own tragedy. Thus also in *Adam Zero* the allegory of a man's life, although it has a wider and more poetic significance than the purely contemporary, seems the more poignant for its shifting symbolic background of modern life and history.

This presentation of a theme in purely imaginative terms is something ballet can achieve in a manner normally outside the scope of the legitimate theatre. Sean O'Casey's war scene in *The Silver Tassie* is its nearest dramatic equivalent and even here the full symbolical and poetical effect was only achieved by the introduction of a balletic stylisation of movement. Auden and Isherwood's use, in their pre-war war play, *On the Frontier*, of a fourth dimension of space into which their lovers, who had never met in life, escaped and communed in their dreams was a device which in terms of dramatic poetry was only partially successful but which suggests endless balletic possibilities.

Both Ashton and Helpmann have used this fourth dimension to suggest a dream atmosphere or mind-projection in their ballets, but its potentialities could be still further explored. The more Freudian psychological traits of the modern individual appear to have been touched on in Antony Tudor's *Pillar of Fire* in America, and they certainly form a part of the spiritual make-up of the moving central figure in Ashton's *The Wanderer*. The problem of the social conditions of the slum, and the gangsterism they breed, has been forcefully suggested in *Miracle in the Gorbals*, but what of the other aspects of modern life and character: the fight for democracy and reconstruction, human despair and spiritual renascence, the *real* English people as distinct from the neurotics, the toughs and the social butterflies? Where in ballet, apart from this one work, can one find the seething humanity of the poor as in Dickens's novels and Sean O'Casey's Dublin tragedies, the earthy callousness and poetic idiom of the peasant as in Synge's *Playboy of the Western World?* A little, perhaps, in the ballets of Soviet Russia and a few by American choreographers; but not, certainly, in the romanticised "noble savages" of *Dark Elegies*, and for all their strength in bereavement Tudor's peasants never achieve the tragic impact of the Irish "keening" in *The Riders to the Sea*.

Social awareness is more alive in the American theatre than our own but it is a quality that penetrates all art in some degree and it is quite distinct from politics in the narrower sense. Henry Moore and Graham Sutherland in art, O'Casey and Clifford Odets in drama, Stephen Spender and Robert Bridges in poetry, Arthur Bliss in such music as his "Morning Heroes," have all reflected the upheavals of our century. Even a genius like Shakespeare, probing to the fundamentals of human character and experience, could not entirely escape the spirit of his own period; it is doubtful how far Hamlet is a portrait of the strange character of Essex, but the play's reflection of the burning spiritualistic and philosophical questions of its day, and its partial debt to Bright's "Treatise of Melancholie," are not now denied.

Ballet, too, is an art vital enough to echo something of the life and spiritual values of its time. "Let us," says Noverre, who can always be guaranteed to put in his oar, "have less of the Fairy Tale, less of the marvellous, more truth and more realism." Much of that truth and that realism has been achieved by Fokine and his successors; but with all the means of imaginative expression at its disposal ballet has still wider potentialities, though it will take the great choreographer to develop them. Mind and human experience in ballet are not elements to be handled by the immature or second-rate; the qualities needed are brain and imagination far more than mere technical facility. Sadler's Wells, by its courage in presenting Helpmann's ballets, has pointed the way and it is for others—including, perhaps, Helpmann himself—to follow and develop ballet's powers as an expression of human life.

CHAPTER XIX

TRENDS IN MODERN BALLET

IF the future of ballet as an art of vitality and importance in the modern world rests to a considerable extent in a broadening and strengthening of its subject material, its ability to consolidate its present achievements to this end, and to create constructively in design and stage production as well as choreography, depends equally on the resources at its disposal and the sound planning of its respective organisations. For this reason the creators of ballet in permanent State-controlled theatres such as those in France and Soviet Russia, and within the Sadler's Wells Company in England, have greater opportunities for achieving constructive and progressive work, if they have the courage and vision to demand and use them, than those in companies formed for commercial purposes by private enterprise, without a consistent policy and frequently disbanding or changing direction and personnel. Certainly this seems to be pointed by conditions in America to-day, where the Russian *émigré* artists who before the war combined to form one strong and productive company, directed by Colonel de Basil, have scattered and become assimilated into various Russian-American companies of uneven quality and by no means assured continuity of existence.

"There are enough good dancers in America to-day," said an American ballet critic to the author in the last year of the war, "to form one really good company." At the time he spoke one recently-formed ballet organisation, after squandering a fortune on production and running a New York season at incredible financial loss, was in the process of paying off its artists, a new company under a different ægis was being planned, and at least two major companies, the Ballet Theatre and the Ballet Russe de Monte Carlo, were contemplating, or had just completed, New York seasons. The vitiation of talent in such circumstances is obvious; and even so some of the best dancers and choreographers in America have been forced fairly frequently, for lack of ballet engagements as much as for financial need, into musical comedy and the films. Individual jealousies and the Russian temperament may play some part in these exclusions, and the need for a fine and disciplined team, including not one but several dancers and choreographers of the "star" class, still seems insufficiently realised.

Without a good permanent company of dancers, whose characteristics and capabilities as individuals and as a team he has had time and opportunity to study, the choreographer is at a disadvantage in creation. This is probably why the English choreographer Antony Tudor, working consistently within the framework of the Ballet Theatre (of which Alicia Markova and Anton Dolin were from its formation in 1940 until 1945 the regular classical "stars" and which has built up behind them a fairly permanent team of dancers) has been able to achieve a more marked personal success than finer and more experienced choreographers, such as Fokine (until his death in 1942), Massine and Nijinska, none of whom, in spite of some successes, seem to have created any ballet of equal choreographic value to their greatest work composed for Russian companies prior to the war. If the mature choreographers have suffered from the "guest-choreographer" and "guest-dancer" system, the young and unfinished talent, such as that of David Lichine—who in the de Basil company, notably with his *Francesca di Rimini*, was beginning to show plastic and dramatic possibilities as a choreographer—has suffered still more through lack of opportunity for regular creative experience and expert guidance at the most important stage of development. Georges Balanchine, attached for some years to the American Ballet at the Metropolitan Opera House in New York, is the only Russian choreographer who has had the benefit of permanent engagement and fairly constant materials on which to work.

Apart from the introduction of some Spanish elements of dance through ballets by Argentinita and her sister Pilar Lopez—well in the tradition of the Russian Ballet which produced Massine's *Tricorne* —and some work, notably *Billy the Kid* and *Rodeo*, of a more distinctive national flavour by Agnes de Mille, ballet in America has carried on intact the Diaghileff–de Basil tradition of lavishness of presentation, fantasy and pure classic dance style with a strong emphasis on pointwork. As a result there has been less an Americanisation of the Russian Ballet than a Russianisation of the American. The strength of the free dance movement in America, led by such strong individual personalities as Martha Graham and Doris Humphreys in the present and Ruth St. Denis in the immediate past, has probably made inevitable a more definite pendulum swing by ballet towards its own technical traditions than, for instance, in England, where ballet has assimilated in certain works some of the characteristics of outside dance movements.

Tudor himself is a choreographer, as his English works have shown, who composes academically in the matter of steps, and the originality to the Americans of his most successful American work, *Pillar of Fire*, as well as of his earlier ballet *Jardin Aux Lilas* (a mainstay of the Ballet Theatre repertoire under the title of *Lilac Garden*), has consisted not in their technique but in their psychological emphasis. His succeeding works, *Romeo and Juliet* and *Dim Lustre*, American critical opinion seems to concur in regarding as ballets, respectively, of decorative beauty and of charm but considerably less effective choreography than *Pillar of Fire*. His *Undertow*, produced in 1945, brings into ballet an exciting new thematic material, the psychology of murder; but its success seems to have been only partial and it aroused considerable controversy in the Press. Nevertheless the repertoire of Tudor works has provided the Ballet Theatre with an original and creative choreographic core which seems lacking from companies which—inspired no doubt by the technical prowess of such dancers as Danilova, Youskewitch, Frederic Franklin or Eglevsky—have concentrated more on the spectacular in the dance and have worked more consistently on the "guest-artist" principle.

Although Markova and Dolin have dominated the classical repertoire other dancers in the company have had opportunities to emerge and develop and in *Pillar of Fire* an American dancer, Nora Kaye, was able to achieve an outstanding dramatic success. Whether the Ballet Theatre will be able to sustain its entity without its two principal classical dancers remains to be seen. The introduction of the beautiful Toumanova, long lost to the films, as guest-ballerina and, according to the estimate of one critic, a technically brilliant misfit, suggested a certain timidity in relying on its own resources as well as a reversion, noticeable also at times on the choreographic side, to the damaging "guest-artist" principle: a system which may eventually ruin America's chances of building a permanent ballet organisation of continuous creative development.[1]

Tudor's *Undertow* has a specially-commissioned score by the

---

[1] The Philadelphia Ballet Company, under the direction of Catherine Littlefield who composed most of the choreography, did continue for some years as an entity with a choreographic and national trend of its own.

American composer William Schuman, one of the few composed for American Ballet since the work of Aaron Copland for Agnes de Mille. It is a point worth noting since the Fokine ideal of close collaboration between choreographer, designer and original musician seems to have been rarely followed in America, where the lack of expert musical guidance, such as the English ballet has had for many years from Constant Lambert, is generally apparent in the choice of existing music for ballet scores. As in France, where Serge Lifar's experiments have been directed towards the complete subservience of the musician to the choreographer, the dance is the predominant factor in Russian-American ballet, although original design seems to have had more artistic encouragement and has even, in the case of a recent Massine ballet designed by the surréalist Salvator Dali, been allowed to overwhelm the choreographic conception.

In Soviet Russia concert composers of the status of Prokofiev and Shostakovich have been encouraged to work in the ballet medium, although Fokine's principles of ballet have only recently begun to influence the academic tradition, which as in all State organisations —perhaps most restrictively of all in the European capitals—is conservatively applied. The four- and five-Act ballet remains the constructive basis. After its first revolutionary experiments under the influence of the constructivist producer Meyerhold, the Russian ballet quickly returned to the basis of pure classicism, and the most important trend since the Revolution has been the infusion into ballet of the rich and diverse national elements of dance to be found among the many races which go to make up the U.S.S.R. Alongside the folk dance and propaganda themes the legendary and the classical have continued to flourish, and the preservation of the former Imperial' Ballet School, with its full traditions of carefully-graded teaching and exhaustive training of dancers, has enabled the technical standard of soloists and *corps de ballet* to be maintained at a higher level of efficiency than are possibly to be found anywhere else in the world. The Soviet ballerinas Ulanova, Semyonova and Lepeshinskaya are, according to their various personalities, in the direct line of succession from Khessinskaya and Préobrajenska of a previous generation, and dancing, rather than choreography, remains the principal genius of the Leningrad and Moscow ballet.

There is no doubt that after thirty years' breakaway from its original centre Russian classicism, both in Russian emigrant and English companies, has lost some of its original style and standards as a result have become confused. Even in Diaghileff's time the restriction of classical ballet to one-Act performances of *Swan Lake* and *Aurora's Wedding* tended slightly to alter the conception of a ballerina as a dancer of lyrical and diamond-hard contrasts, and to give the dancing of the second Act of the first ballet a colder and harder style than would have been possible had the dancer had to follow it with the contrasting virtuosity of the third Act. The *danseur noble* was seen also in these circumstances only in his capacities as *porteur* and dancer, and his equally essential function as a mime was not realised until the performances of Robert Helpmann in the full-length versions of *Lac des Cygnes* and *The Sleeping Beauty* revealed the absolute necessity of mimic ability in the dancer to carry the dramatic action forward through the long passages of sign language. Perfect classical style, a matter of natural dignity, musicality and intelligence as well as of balance and line in the carriage of torso, head and arms, is becoming increasingly rare; and the speeding up of the training of the dancer, justified to some extent though it may be by the increase of anatomical knowledge, tends to slur over these essentials of style and to start the dancer well on her career before absolute control and precision have been attained. Under modern conditions of constant rehearsal, travelling and performance such defects, once the dancer has taken her place in a company, are extremely difficult to eradicate and the problem of the brilliantly promising young dancer who after two or three years has not only failed to progress, but has actually begun to deteriorate, is an urgent one in English companies.

In Russia the schooling of the dancer is so graded that she has the teacher exactly suited to her particular stage of development throughout the training period, beginning with the teacher whose particular flair is for the instillation of technical groundwork and ending with the one whose greatest value is in the advanced work of the "perfection class." This is an ideal not yet realised over here, although the best dancers, like the great Russians Pavlova and Karsavina before them, understand quickly enough the need for increasing their variety and strength through lessons with various teachers. Both Margot Fonteyn and Robert Helpmann, the most finished stylists among English dancers to-day, have studied with a number of teachers, including the Russians Astafieva, Legat, Préobrajenska and Vera Volkova in the first case and Novikoff, Préobrajenska and Volkova in the second. Moira Shearer, one of the most outstandingly promising of English classical dancers, was a pupil of Nadine Nicolaeva-Legat. Alexis

Rassine, British by nationality although Russian-Lithuanian by parentage and birth, studied with Préobrajenska, Gordon Hamilton with Egorova, Harold Turner with Nicholas Legat and Marie Rambert (whose system of teaching, however, approximates more to the Cecchetti or Italian school). The list might be prolonged, but enough has been written to make it obvious that the work of the English teacher (and owing to the careful system of control of the Royal Academy of Dancing, founded by Adeline Genée, teaching of the dance in England is of a generally good standard) is frequently supplemented by direct contact with the Russian school on which English classic technique is still basically founded. The appointment into the Sadler's Wells Ballet School of Vera Volkova, an exceptionally gifted teacher and ex-dancer of the Soviet Ballet who herself was trained in the Leningrad School, brings English dancers into still closer contact with the original Russian "style" and technique.

A national ballet school should command the services of the finest teachers available, and there is a special need for a good male teacher, if only for instruction in "double-work," the absence of which in the past may account for the generally low standard of partnering (and therefore of the alarming lack of true *danseurs noble*) among English dancers. The particular values of Volkova's teaching are her concentration on the most subtle details of style, *épaulement* and alignment, on the position of every limb and her insistence, even in class *enchaînements*, on a fluidity and grace of movement, allied with attack, that reduces the possibility, if the idea is assimilated by the dancer, of classroom technicalities being transferred too obviously on to the stage.

If, however, as is now realised, general artistic education is important as well as dance training in the development of the ballet artist (especially bearing in mind that it is from the ranks of dance students that the choreographer of the future must spring),the ideal is for general and stage education to be combined in the school curriculum. The allocation of time for each subject can then be planned so that the dancer may absorb the knowledge which will have the most beneficial effect, direct or indirect, on her future, and at the same time acquire the mental alertness and sensibility to beauty without which no dancer is likely to rise above the merely competent. This comprehensive system of education has always been maintained in the Russian State School, both under the Czar and the Soviet, and it was already being planned by the Sadler's Wells School when the war temporarily interrupted all such developments. In England, outside Sadler's Wells, it has been adopted intact for some years by the Legat School, where the students are educated to Oxford School Certificate and Matriculation standard and are trained by Madame Legat in the pure classical style of the Russian 'Imperial Ballet, which derives from the great teacher Johannsen and was first taught in England by her husband, the late Nicholas Legat.

The Russian school of dance absorbed everything it could learn from the French and Italian schools and then fashioned the materials anew in its own image, with a different line, *épaulement* and execution of steps and arm movements, and the infusion of dramatic feeling into dance as well as mime. It is on this Russian school that the English is founded, and since the Russian classical ballets form the foundation-stone of the repertoire it is right that it should be so. But in the creation of its own ballets the Sadler's Wells Ballet is already showing the development of a more eclectic style, drawing in a ballet such as *Dante Sonata* on Central European influences and evolving in such works as *Job*, *The Rake's Progress*, *Hamlet* and *Miracle in the Gorbals* (which achieved a sensational success, shared equally by *The Rake's Progress*, in Paris, the European centre of critical knowledge and classic traditions) an individual blend of drama, characterisation and movement which makes all four ballets indefinably but characteristically "English."

"Car si le ballet français était avant tout le ballet des pointes et des entrechats," wrote the critic of *Le Monde Illustré* in March 1945, "si le ballet russe a triomphé en tant que fête de la fantaisie, de la fantasmagorie, de la saltation dionysiaque, ce ballet anglais trouve son caractère et sa qualité dans la souplesse et la variété de sa discipline, dans l'art d'équilibrer l'action dansée et mimée, et dans l'art non moins remarquable d'employer des moyens très discrets, des inflexions chorégraphique parfois presque imperceptibles."   It is this feeling for "l'art d'équilibrer l'action dansée et mimée" which makes the Sadler's Wells Ballet a choreographic force that becomes at times a truly national expression. If standards of choreography, the creative elements, are the true measure of a ballet company's worth and powers of survival—and I maintain that they are—the Sadler's Wells Ballet is in an unrivalled position in England and possibly in the world to-day; in direct line of succession, in spite of the differences of style and national colour, to the Diaghileff Ballet of the Fokine period, as more than one French and Belgian critic was quick to recognise.

It is the lack of high standards of new choreography, in addition to a lavishness of production which in the case of ballets such as

Giselle has tended to destroy the atmosphere and subtlety of the work, that has prevented the International Ballet from taking the place in war-time ballet history to which some of the individual dancing (several of the finest Sadler's Wells soloists came from this company) might have entitled it. Its director, Mona Inglesby, is herself a fluent classical dancer, lacking in expression and attack but with a fine arabesque line, grace and musicality; but as a choreographer, in spite of occasional beauty of grouping in the style of the mediæval frieze, she lacks a sense of drama, expressiveness in characterisation, and that pattern and fluidity of movement without which the groupings become meaningless.

The Anglo-Polish Ballet, more individual in style, began better with two dynamic Polish dancers, Alicja Halama and Cz. Konarski, and a small but lively repertoire of ballets in which Konarski, as choreographer, made some charming use of Polish dance material. *Cracow Wedding, Matthew is Dead* and the acrobatic *Dancing Woman*, brilliantly performed by the lean, lissom and beautiful Halama, had a humour, gauche but original, of their own; and in *Pan Twardowski*, although the treatment of the Faust theme lacked dramatic form and the Polish dances were repetitive and uninventive, Konarski achieved a Hell Scene of startling rhythmic and resurgent force. When Halama and Konarski left the company lost immeasurably in verve and cohesion and subsisted on a dwindling repertoire of ballets and *divertissement*. It will not take a serious position in the English ballet scene unless it regains its original choreographer and principal dancers and develops a fresh and individualistic choreography while re-vitalising the old. Outside these companies and the miniaturist Ballet Rambert, far more important in choreography and integrity of direction, there are several practising choreographers, including Wendy Toye and the musical dancer Pauline Grant, whose work within the musical comedy machine is too hampered by lack of the right atmosphere and materials, and by its own impermanency, to come within the proper boundaries of English ballet.

The Sadler's Wells Company has this precious gift of permanency and full resources of development as the English national ballet. It has had, and gives every indication of continuing to produce, a fine selection of dramatic mimes, without whom some of its most indi-vidualistic ballets, notably those of Ninette de Valois and Robert Helpmann, could not have been effectively produced. There is enough dancing talent of good classical style, some of it not yet seriously tapped, to suggest considerable hope for the future if it is adequately cast and directed, and the return of male dancers from the Forces should make possible a finer balance in the classical ballets between ballerina, *premier danseur* and the remaining company, and facilitate the revival of some old ballets, as well as the production of new ones, in which both the male and female *corps de ballet* are exploited to enhance the richness of the dance orchestration. *Horoscope, Checkmate, Apparitions* and *The Wanderer* have been for too long periods absent from this company's repertoire, and part of their splendour is in this contrast and harmony of masculine and feminine movement.

The Wanderer will be a testpiece of this company's post-war æsthetic policy just because, although a superb work with a particular appeal to many balletgoers, it was less generally popular than most large-scale works and rarely drew a full house.[1] But if the Sadler's Wells Company is truly to function as a national ballet it must be prepared, as the Old Vic Drama Company has had to be prepared, to "carry" a few works by outstanding English creators on their artistic and historic value, irrespective of commercial considerations. A national drama and ballet should be a repository for the preservation of fine plays and ballets; it is a national trust, and the need for fairly frequent revival is more urgent in the case of ballet since ballets cannot be written down and preserved on paper but must be reconstructed from the living memory of those who created or took part in them. Strictly speaking the national heritage in ballet consists not only in the ballets performed by Sadler's Wells but in the best works of all English choreographers, and a true historic record would consist of Ashton ballets such as *Capriol Suite* and *Mephisto Valse*, both produced for the Ballet Rambert and important examples of the choreographer's formative period, as well as a ballet such as Tudor's *Jardin Aux Lilas*. None of these ballets need be restricted to the chamber ballet medium; the Tudor work has, as has been seen, already been performed on a large stage in America and in *Mephisto Valse* the choreographic movement of the three couples of the *corps de ballet* as they now exist is so complex and striking that only the addition of several more couples is necessary to turn this ballet, as the choreographer himself would wish, into a full-scale work. The necessity for the inclusion of modern foreign classics as well as those of the past in a representative and educational repertoire is already realised, and Massine's *La Boutique*

[1] Its revival at Sadler's Wells Theatre in 1945 suggested it had a much stronger appeal to the new ballet audience, but too few performances were given to test this impression.

Fantasque is one of the ballets suggested for future production. Invitations to famous foreign choreographers to work with Sadler's Wells for a period and mount ballets on the company were also contemplated at the outbreak of war, and the eclecticism of outlook of the director was shown by the issue of a similar invitation, which was not accepted, to Kurt Jooss.

The encouragement of new choreographers from within the company will be more possible now Sadler's Wells has been able to create a second company; this was a necessity if the large provincial audience for ballet which has been evolved since the war is to be catered for in addition to the London one. There is a need, while preserving mature choreographic standards in the principal company, for an experimental outlet for the untrained choreographer; such an outlet has always been provided by the Ballet Rambert but the dancer already within Sadler's Wells can have no opportunity for choreographic training unless the organisation itself provides the opportunities.

With the access to more varied resources and materials through scientific experiment after the war there will be new potentialities in stage production which ballet, by its concentration on the visual and its power to express the symbolic through the medium of an imagined fourth dimension, is by its nature particularly fitted to exploit. Artists have already realised the chameleonlike possibilities of plastics in the building of theatrical *décor* and if the substance can be strengthened —it is at present inclined to brittleness—to withstand the necessary hard wear and tear of scene-shifting and touring, its transparency and malleability in the creation of forms and surfaces, especially if heightened by effects of lighting, could be used to create ballet *décor* of great suggestibility and beauty.

Ballet in recent years has inclined to the conventional in design and except in the case of the ballets of Kurt Jooss and Robert Helpmann, both of whom think of lighting as an integral part of the dramatic action, lighting has never played more than a very subsidiary part. Certainly ballet has never again used it as an equal partner in the choreographic composition as it was used in the Diaghileff production of Massine's *Ode*, when plastic pictures were evolved purely through the medium of coloured light, very much in the tradition of the American dancer Loie Fuller, who in the last years of the nineteenth century made experiments in light, prismatic, phosphorescent and in relation to coloured materials of various textures, which formed the essence of her dance and achieved pictorial effects of such beauty and originality that the sculptor Rodin acknowledged her genius. Stage production becomes a danger when it is used to gloss over the choreographic or dramatic paucity beneath it; but it may still be used as an enhancement of the creator's theme or composition, and it is extraordinary that the experimental ideas of Gordon Craig, a genius the English dramatic theatre has dismissed as impracticable, should not have more influenced ballet production. The subtle psychological atmosphere and suggestion of his Moscow production of *Hamlet* appear to have shown a balletic rather than a dramatic approach and his theories, imaginatively applied, might still provide a rich creative impulse to the choreographer and designer of ballet.

If ballet, however, is going to make full use of such methods of lighting and production it must provide themes adaptable to such treatment. Ballet—and this applies to the realistic *ballet d'action* as well as to that less definitive in theme—needs good scenarists as well as good choreographers and both are rare. The poet Boris Kochno, scenarist of Balanchine's *Cotillon*, and Constant Lambert have provided excellent themes for ballet and the recent emergence of Michael Benthall, author of *Miracle in the Gorbals* and *Adam Zero* as well as of a very fine ballet adaptation, subsequently abandoned by the choreographer, of Wilde's *Picture of Dorian Gray*, brings an interesting new mind, at once sensitive and forceful, into English ballet. Benthall's experience as an actor before the war has given him a dramatic sense completely in key with the natural style of ballet in England, as well as providing an effective basis on which the choreographer for whom he writes, Robert Helpmann, may embroider the vivid tapestry of his characterisation. His impressionability to contemporary life—*Miracle in the Gorbals* was conceived during his period in Glasgow, as a Captain of the Royal Artillery, prior to the invasion of the Continent, and *Adam Zero*, as originally drafted, showed the influence of the war devastation of his surroundings while on active service in Holland—may be an important influence in the future. The last ballet is not merely a remarkable morality which required exceptional powers of imaginative composition in the choreographer (for the scenario, important though it is, provides only the bare skeleton of ballet on which the choreographer must build the flesh and living tissue), it is a theme which could only have been realised in terms of the most inventive production and design. For the creation of such progressive work a large theatre is an essential, and English ballet is now of an international importance that justifies its appearance in the theatre at which the greatest foreign opera and ballet companies have performed. Covent Garden not only gives English ballet new opportunities to spread its wings, it will encourage a lease-lend system of exchange with the greatest companies abroad, and help to dispel the isolationism into which all branches of the English theatre have been forced by six years of war.

The visit of Les Ballets des Champs-Élysées to the Adelphi Theatre in April 1946 was the first rift in this isolationism and gave us our first opportunity since before the war to compare the artistic standards of an English and foreign company. English ballet did not suffer by the comparison, especially in respect of its choreographic achievement, its discipline and its standard of execution and production in the classics. But if the young French company, scarcely a year old, lacked a sense of teamwork, and placed too much emphasis on the mechanics of technique and too little on "line" and expression, it had abundant vitality and promise, and under the artistic direction of Boris Kochno, with *décor* by artists such as Christian Bérard and music by Stravinsky and Ibert, it showed a genuine desire to break away from some Paris Opera traditions and to create ballet along the Diaghileff lines of artistic unity. It also possessed some male dancers of unusual excellence, of whom Jean Babilée and Roland Petit were outstanding, and in Petit a *maître de ballet*, choreographer, *danseur noble* and mime of a quality and maturity of style quite remarkable in one so young.

Petit's ballets were the mainstay of the repertoire; as a choreographer he has imagination, invention and drama, and although his work is uneven and tends at times to acrobacy for its own sake, in *Les Forains* at least he has produced a ballet of perfect consistency and magical charm.

This impression of a small and weary band of gypsies, who set up their circus "props" and give a performance in which they acquire a sudden joyous and evanescent glitter, take the hat round in vain and once again push their wagon dejectedly on to the road again, has in it the heartache, tawdriness and tinsel glamour of all nomad theatrical life. There is mime and expression here as well as dance, and with music of sparkling tunefulness by Henri Sauguet and designs by Bérard the ballet catches at the heart as well as the senses. It gained much from Petit's own intensely sympathetic performance as leader of the troupe, and established the company as one of rich creative possibilities. Already it is producing a style of its own. But the fact that on its departure it took with it one of the most talented and intelligent of Sadler's Wells dancers and mimes, Gordon Hamilton, awakened one to the uneasy realisation that the eagerly-awaited visits of foreign companies to these shores may prove, as far as English ballet is concerned, a two-edged sword.

Every ballet organisation that has had any significance in the history of the art has had something of its own to give, a style, a feeling, an atmosphere that is recognisable to itself. It seems fairly certain that English ballet will continue to develop on mimeodramatic lines and Russian Ballet, as in the past, on those of spectacle, fantasy and glamour. Let the final tribute to a more recent dramatic achievement of English ballet, and summing up of its characteristics, be that of an intelligent and impartial foreign critic, Guillot de Rode, whose article in the Parisian paper *Action* on 23rd March 1945 I quote in full:

"Les quelques lignes élogieuses consacrées de-ci, de-là aux ballets anglais se contentent de les comparer aux ballets russes et demeurent d'autant plus insuffisantes que cet éloge qui risque de leur causer plus de mal que de bien: il ne met nullement en lumière leur originalité profonde.

"En effet, les reprises qu'ils présentent, comme *Sylphides* ou surtout *Carnaval*, ne sont pas parfaites et ne révèlent pas du tout le style d'une troupe dont le ressort profond n'est pas celui de la danse academique traditionnelle. La magistrale exécution, par Margot Fonteyn et Robert Helpmann, du pas de deux célèbre de *Casse Noisette*, aussi bien que les vingt-neuf fouettés de tel sujet dans *Patineurs*, prouvent assez la valeur de la troupe en fait de technique d'école et la connaissance de disciplines et de règles que ses chorégraphes n'utilisent ou ne violent qu'à bon escient. Parmi nombre de créations interéssantes comme *The Rake's Progress* ou la magnifique et poignante *Dante Sonata*, il convient de fair une place toute spéciale à une oeuvre de très grande classe: *Miracle in the Gorbals* (musique de Arthur Bliss). Certainement l'une des meilleures réussites chorégraphiques de notre époque, ce ballet réaliste dont l'action se situe dans un quartier populeux des bords de la Clyde, dégage d'un bout à l'autre une puissance émotive d'une densité extraordinaire. Revolutionnaire et mystique, grouillant et dépouillé, pur et amer, son style évoque inconsciemment celui du cinéma soviétique de la grand époque et les meilleures réalisations de Kurt Jooss. Au travers de mouvements de foule excellents, les tableaux se succèdent avec une science étonnante de la composition, de l'éclairage, de l'atmosphère. D'un sujet dangereux à souhait et rempli d'embûches, le chorégraphe a su tirer une oeuvre magnifique de la vérité dramatique et d'intensité poétique.

"L'interprétation est parfaite. Robert Helpmann y crée en particulier une figure inoubliable. Dans ce ballet plus encore que dans d'autres où nous l'avions déjà remarquée apparait la splendide discipline de cette troupe jeune et homogène, en plein progrès, où l'on sent constamment l'amour de l'oeuvre créée et la foi en l'art servi."

CHAPTER XX

THE AUDIENCE AND THE CRITIC

TWO factors in the creation of a progressive and vital art of ballet have not been previously considered in this book: the audience and the critic. Their influence is purely external and where the creative urge of the artists is strong and original ballet will follow its artistic course and, if necessary, carry out its reforms irrespective of outside criticism and judgment. Nevertheless an intelligent, responsive and broadminded audience, free from both hysteria and intellectual snobbery, is a necessity if the work of the artist is not to be hampered and his freedom of expression achieved without bitterness and conflict. Unfortunately in England to-day this balance of outlook between audience and critic on the one hand, and choreographer and dancer on the other, only partially exists; much of the audience tends to be more of a hindrance than a help to ballet creation, its attitude ranging, according to its personal bias and length of experience, from destructive criticism to a hysterical partisanship of individual artists that is a continual source of irritation to the serious-minded artist.

Partly, of course, this is the result of the phenomenal increase in popularity of ballet since the war, the introduction of a new large audience of indiscriminate enthusiasm and no critical standards having lashed the more dissatisfied elements of greater experience into an opposite extreme of derogation. In neither case is the mentality adult, and the fact that the second type frequently springs from a previous generation of the "lunatic fringe" appears to add to the viciousness of the criticisms made.

There is no derogation more unbalanced and malicious than that of the ballet partisan who has turned turtle, especially when it springs, as frequently happens, from personal animosity towards a particular artist or company, and most editors who number a ballet critic among their contributors, and the critics themselves, will at some period have been the recipients of letters from this particular pathological type. Such manifestations would not be worth commenting on if it were

not for the fact that they occasionally find their way into print—
amateur criticism, sometimes overlapping into the professional, has
considerably extended in scope since the war—and for the unfortunate
effect on the artist, who quite naturally thereafter inclines to take a
cynical view of praise and blame and to hide his hurt (and the theatre
artist is generally most hurt when he is most apparently contemptuous
of criticism) in a dangerous mistrust of the value of all criticism.
Obvious injustice damages the prestige of all critics and in ballet,
where the critic frequently comes from the audience and where, owing
to the complexity of the subject, critical comment is very often based
on that little knowledge that is a dangerous thing, the taint can be
serious. Certainly the ballet critic in England cannot avoid feeling,
at times, his superfluity in the eyes of the artist.[1]

Fortunately this is not the whole picture, and the fact that the
unbalanced minority of the audience is the more vocal and obstrusive
causes its importance, at times, to be exaggerated out of all proportion
to its size. The gallery and upper circle are not synonymous with the
audience, although they tend to become so in many minds, and it is
possible to sit in another part of the theatre among onlookers dis-
criminately withholding their applause while the gallery is still
clamouring for a dancer to take a fourth bow after a not very notable
variation. It is a depressing reflection for the socialist that balletic
taste does superficially appear to vary to some extent according to
income, although in actual fact this is less a matter of social class
than of age. The earnings of the youth of all classes are comparatively
low and the gallerygoer of to-day is frequently the stallholder of
to-morrow. By the time this migration has taken place he has normally
reached years of discretion; although the difficulty of obtaining seats
in the war-time "boom" has tended to accelerate the progress from
gallery to stalls, probably at the expense of a sharp rise in the percentage
of youthful bankrupts as well as a corresponding decrease in the
average age of the stalls and dress circle audience.

Nevertheless it is a mistake to assume that hysteria in applause and
abuse is as widespread as would superficially appear even among the
younger and newer elements in the audience, and length of experience
is not necessarily a guarantee of critical taste, which is at least to some
extent inborn. Anyone who has lectured, as I have done regularly
during the last few years, to theatre groups, A.T.S. Units and L.C.C.

[1] "Books on ballet ought never to be written!" cried a sufferer to the author,
with notable sincerity if not exactly with tact.

evening institute students, must be aware of a serious interest and desire to learn among a proportion of balletgoers, and the interest is by no means confined to present-day dancers and performances, although in the large majority of cases the listeners have seen no others. Ballet Clubs in the provinces and London have also fomented a more knowledgeable interest and as long as those banes of amateur theatricalism, self-complacency and depreciation of the professional, do not unbalance the members' view of the art as a whole these will play a large part in forming the audience of the future. Certainly the intelligent and critically sober letters received by the critic outnumber those of the opposite variety, and occasionally they give an interesting insight into the formative-process that goes to make a balletgoer:

"A year ago," began one such letter, "I had never been to a ballet. Various people had tried to persuade me but I maintained the perverse and prejudiced attitude so prevalent among the general public. Ever since I can remember the theatre has been the most important thing in my life, and I just could not accept ballet as a part of theatre tradition any more than I am yet able to accept opera. Then I happened to read one of your articles on the Sadler's Wells Company in *Theatre World*. I was interested. I turned up all my old copies and read all the articles you had written, and found myself experiencing an intense desire to pay a visit to the ballet.

"The first ballet I ever saw was *The Rake's Progress*. Everything you had written came to life before my eyes. I was totally ignorant of any technical knowledge of dancing, but I was in no doubt about Helpmann's performance. I went again and again, first to see him act, then to concentrate on the actual dancing and later to be able to appreciate the whole. It may seem a very roundabout way, but I got there at last."

Apart from its suggestion that the critic may hold a certain responsibility as a propaganda force, the interesting point about this letter is the recognition that the final stage of the balletgoer's development is the ability to appreciate the work *as a whole*. Some balletgoers never reach this stage, but its necessity is increasingly realised, as other letters have shown. The most intelligent appreciation of the true function of criticism in ballet came from a member of the Manchester Ballet Club, who wrote:

"Surely the function of the critic is to criticise the choreography, *décor* and music (individual performances coming last), to say whether any new movement has been added to the technique and to judge if the theme has been sympathetically treated. In most criticism I can think of too much emphasis is laid on the actual performance, not on the ballet as a complete work of art."

The reaction against personality-emphasis in ballet has resulted in a school of thought which would go to the opposite extreme and leave out mention of performances altogether: an ideal which is suspect not only because the capacity to judge the merits of a performance is an integral part of the function of a ballet as of a dramatic critic, but because in practice it has been operated to enforce a bias against certain artists. It is obvious, since the dancer is the indispensable tool of the choreographer, that ballet will not progress as an art if the tools the choreographer must use are defective; standards of critical judgment in respect of dancing and acting performance are therefore as essential as choreographic standards in the critic, and in practice it is unfortunately true that the regular writer on ballet will be forced, on occasion, to concentrate more on performances than ballets owing to the lack of new productions to review. The position is the same as that of the dramatic critic who, faced with his tenth or twelfth production of *Hamlet*, can find little fresh to say about the play except insofar as new angles of it may be revealed through the performance of the actor.

Ballet criticism in England suffers a serious handicap through the fact that it is not a recognised speciality in the average newspaper or magazine, but is dealt with by the drama, film or music critic, who attends performances too infrequently ("press" nights cover only a modicum of the ballets which comprise one company's repertoire) to have acquired any serious evaluations, and who has, generally speaking and unlike his foreign *confrère*, made no intimate study of choreography or of dance.[1] The late Edwin Evans, a music critic who had worked with Diaghileff and had a real knowledge of ballet, was one of the few exceptions. It is a comment, perhaps, on the position of ballet as an art in this country that even in the Critics' Circle, where

[1] The fact that the management of a major English company invites reporters and gossip-writers to its First Nights but excludes the critic who writes seriously and at length on the subject does not, however, encourage one to feel that attempts to raise the status of ballet criticism will meet with any sympathy or support within ballet circles. And it must be noted that in any case the infrequency of new productions and "press" nights, and the expense involved in attending other performances (ballets can only be studied in the theatre), make ballet criticism at best a precarious and unrewarding profession.

there are separate sections for Drama, Music and the Films, the ballet critic as such has no recognition but is absorbed into the Music Section. There is no reason why the music critic—or equally the dramatic or art critic—should not be a ballet critic of distinction and it is an undeniable fact that the freedom of such critics from any of the personal bias and "isms" that infect internal ballet politics, and their broader sense of values acquired through the judgment of great work in their own subject, does enable them sometimes to recognise instinctively the quality of a work which the critic who is the direct product of balletomania, and obsessed with technical details, will miss. But instinct without knowledge is not good enough, and I suspect it was with something more than instinct that, twenty years before the work of Fokine was seen in Europe and ten before he began serious creation, a young music and dramatic critic, George Bernard Shaw, was writing in a review of an Alhambra ballet performance that ballet should be "a whole drama in dance, in which the *pas seul* shall merge, as the aria and cavatina have at last merged in the Wagnerian music–drama." "In opera," he pointed out, "this has been done by a gradual reduction of the independence and consequent incongruity of the soloist's show-piece until it became an integral part of the act. But I cannot say that I see much progress in this direction in the ballet." There follows a dissertation on criticism that still might be absorbed with profit by the balletomane:

"The very vilest phase of criticism is that in which it emerges from blank inanity into an acquaintance with the terms, rules, and superstitions which belong to the technical processes of the art treated of. It is then that you get asinine rigmaroles praising hopelessly commonplace painters for their 'marvellous fore-shortening,' their knowledge of anatomy, their 'correct composition' (meaning that every group of figures has the outline of a candle extinguisher), and so on; whilst great composers are proved to be ignorant and tasteless pretenders, because their discords are unprepared and improperly resolved, or their harmony full of false relations and consecutive fifths, or because *si contra fa diabolus est*. Why, I have myself been reproached with ignorance of 'the science of music' because I do not impose on the public by hoggishly irrelevant displays of ignorance of the true inwardness of musical technology! Now it happens that in an evil hour the technology of the ballet has been betrayed to the critics by a friend of mine. Being a clergyman,[1] he found it

---

[1] Rev. Stewart Headlam.

necessary to disabuse his clients of their pious opinion that a ballet-dancer is a daughter of Satan who wears short skirts in order that she may cut lewd capers. He bore eloquent testimony to the devoted labour and perseverance involved by the training of a fine dancer, and declared his conviction of the perfect godliness of high art in that and all other forms. To this day you may see in the list of his works the title 'Art of Theatrical Dancing,' immediately following 'Laws of Eternal Life.' All this is much to his credit; but unfortunately his indiscreet revelation of how a critic with no artistic sense of dancing may cover up his incapacity by talking about *ronds de jambe*, arabesques, elevation, *entrechats, ballonnés*, and the like, threatens to start a technico-jargonautic fashion in ballet criticism, and whilst it lasts there will be no abolishing the absurdities and pedantries which now hamper the development of stage-dancing."

Ballet in modern times as in the past has suffered from the type of criticism which cannot see the wood for the trees and will damn the work of a new and vital mentality on the ground that it breaks the rules the critic has laid down. But the great artist will always break rules; they are too narrow for his mind, and it can be safely said that had choreographers in the past listened to the innumerable "don'ts" of the balletomanes and critics of their time ballet as an art would long since have cancelled itself out by a process of negation.

Nevertheless free and constructive criticism, impartially applied to all artists and companies, is a necessity if criticism is to have any value or point at all, and unfortunately in ballet the propagandist, rather than the true critic, is on the increase. The Critics' Circle has a very good rule that no critic shall be allowed to continue as a member if he is associated in any way with publicity work; a rule devised to keep the profession of criticism on the highest level of incorruptibility. In England ballet criticism has had, in the last twenty years, a traditional association with Press representative and publicity work and although in one or two cases it has not obviously affected the fairness of the critic's judgment the danger is obvious. The more recent type of unpaid propagandist, the ballet "fan" with an axe to grind on behalf of a favourite company, is often a more serious menace since while withholding all criticism from this particular company he will sometimes unscrupulously apply it to others. It is easy to see, in the circumstances, why the director of the major English ballet company, which has suffered a good deal from this type of *coterie* criticism, should have made a rule, rigorously applied, that no writer on ballet may attend classes or rehearsals or in any way penetrate into the ballet "workshop"; although there is no doubt that lack of opportunities for first-hand study which were the prerogative of ballet critics, Russian and French, in the past is a handicap to the serious critic wishing not merely to review performances but to write with a thorough internal knowledge of every aspect of ballet creation, choreographic as well as dancing. The degree of contact and conversation with artists, both creative and interpretative, is a problem the critic must eventually solve for himself, and much of interest can be learned in this way if the critic keeps his mind open to all points of view and realises the vital truth that the artist's judgments will almost inevitably be coloured to some extent by his own natural instincts and ideals. In ballet as in other arts there are many ways of being right. It is only the bad, or very young, critic who lets what he hears behind-scenes or a personal friendship influence his final judgment of the work seen from the auditorium.

The prestige of an art is enhanced by the prestige of its critics; and in Paris, that city of jealously-guarded ballet traditions where the critic has still a position of some authority and the art of ballet is considered important enough to be allotted a review space unheard of in this country, the Sadler's Wells Ballet inspired a fine selection of knowledgeable criticisms which grasped the essence of English ballet with a breadth of outlook and sensibility to new styles rarely met with in writing on the English national ballet in its own country. "The critic," wrote Oscar Wilde, "is he who can translate into another manner or a new material his impression of beautiful things." Dramatic and ballet criticism represent, like playwriting, the literary side of the theatre; acting and dancing the interpretative side. The critic is, potentially and at his best, an artist; an artist not creative but analytic and descriptive, with words as his instruments of expression. It is only when this is recognised by the artists within ballet and by English editors that criticism in England will become worthy of its subject and ballet itself achieve the status accorded in some journals to drama, music and the films.

In view of the tendency of so much that is written on ballet in England to-day it is worth reiterating that no criticism worthy the name is ever purely destructive or written to suggest the cleverness of the critic at the expense of the artist, and catholicism of taste, together with a sympathetic awareness of the problems of the creative artist in his struggle for individual expression, are essential if ballet is to be a progressive art with a wide variety of styles and mental vigour. It is inevitable that the critic, who is human, will have personal preferences, but they should not be allowed to affect his critical judgment where the work is good of its kind. The best criticism proceeds not from the desire to censure but from the desire to salute and analyse a fine achievement: Hazlitt on Kean and Lamb on Munden are more important than Leigh Hunt on the actor Pope, who tore "a passion to tatters, to very rags."

> "A perfect Judge will read each work of Wit
> With the same spirit that its author writ:
> Survey the WHOLE, nor seek slight faults to find
> Where nature moves, and rapture warms the mind;
> Nor lose, for that malignant dull delight,
> The gen'rous pleasure to be charm'd with wit."

Thus Alexander Pope in his *Essay on Criticism*, and he merely put into verse what every serious critic, from Carlyle to Agate, has recognised and pointed out in prose. Probably for this reason, the underlying need for love of the art criticised, some of the most constructive and objective criticism has been written by artists of the theatre themselves. William Poel, Granville-Barker, Stanislavsky in the drama, Noverre, Fokine, in modern times Karsavina in *Theatre Street* and Ninette de Valois in *Invitation to the Ballet*, have achieved an objectivity of outlook and balanced understanding of their art unmatched in the work of the average outside critic. Their work remains an indispensable guide to the study of their art and every critic of drama and ballet (and I speak in both capacities) must acknowledge a debt to them. The future of ballet is still in the hands of the creative artists, and the foundation on which they must build the vision of Noverre and Fokine which places ballet on a level of expression and power with its corollary arts of drama, painting and music.

London.
1945–6.

INDEX